Handbook
Cardiac Catheterisation

GRAHAM A. H. MILLER
MA, BSc, DM, FRCP
Formerly
Consultant Cardiologist and Director
Cardiac Laboratories
Brompton Hospital
London

BLACKWELL SCIENTIFIC PUBLICATIONS

OXFORD LONDON

EDINBURGH BOSTON MELBOURNE

© 1990 by
Blackwell Scientific Publications
Editorial Offices:
Osney Mead, Oxford OX2 0EL
25 John Street, London WC1N 2BL
23 Ainslie Place, Edinburgh EH3 6AJ
3 Cambridge Center, Suite 208,
    Cambridge, Massachusetts 02142,
    USA
107 Barry Street, Carlton
    Victoria 3053, Australia

First published 1990

Set in Palatino and Helvetica by
Setrite Typesetters, Hong Kong
Printed and bound in Great Britain
by The Alden Press, Oxford

DISTRIBUTORS

Marston Book Services Ltd
PO Box 87
Oxford OX2 0DT
(*Orders*: Tel: 0865 791155
         Fax: 0865 791927
         Telex: 837515

USA
Year Book Medical Publishers
200 North LaSalle Street
Chicago, Illinois 60601
(*Orders*: Tel: (312) 726−9733)

Canada
The C.V. Mosby Company
5240 Finch Avenue East
Scarborough, Ontario
(*Orders*: Tel: (416) 298−1588)

Australia
Blackwell Scientific Publications
(Australia) Pty Ltd
107 Barry Street
Carlton, Victoria 3053
(*Orders*: Tel: (03) 347−0300)

British Library
Cataloguing in Publication Data

Miller, Graham, A.H.
    Handbook of cardiac
    catheterisation.
    1. Man. Heart. Diagnosis.
    Catheterisation
    I. Title
    616.1'20754

ISBN 0−632−02691−X

Contents

Preface

I have written this *Handbook of Cardiac Catheterisation* in the belief that there is a need for a short text that explains why and how catheterisation is performed. It is addressed to students and junior doctors who are meeting cardiology for the first time and who need to understand the basic principles but do not need the detailed information provided in larger and more expensive textbooks. It is my hope that this short text will also be of use to nurses caring for cardiac patients, and to the nurses, technicians and radiographers who play an essential part in the catheterisation laboratory, but may not always understand why a certain procedure is being performed or the significance of the results obtained.

The technique of cardiac catheterisation has been an essential part of the diagnostic 'work-up' of most patients with heart disease since the 1940s. It still is. Many of those working in cardiology were first attracted to the subject because catheterisation provided an unequivocal diagnostic test and because performing cardiac catheterisation required technical skill. Catheterisation is an 'invasive' procedure involving a (very) small risk and a small degree of discomfort for the patient. Catheterisation should not be performed, therefore, if an alternative 'non-invasive' investigation can provide all the information needed for the patient's management. Nor should the procedure be prolonged in pursuit of further information when that information will not affect what is best done for the patient. Conversely, a patient is ill-served by a 'non-invasive' investigation that provides incomplete or equivocal information; catheterisation is then indicated and it is the operator's responsibility to ensure that everything is done to minimise the risk and to bring the procedure to a swift and painless conclusion, while still obtaining all the essential information. It is not only the operator who is involved; the nursing staff can allay the patient's understandable anxiety by explaining the procedure, and smooth teamwork in the laboratory — technicians, radiographers, nurses and cardiologists — all contribute to a safe and speedy study. It has been my privilege to work with such a team at the Brompton Hospital and I take this opportunity to acknowledge my enormous debt to them all.

Graham A.H. Miller, 1989

Introduction — a short history of cardiac catheterisation

In 1929 Werner Forssmann, in Germany, became the first to introduce a catheter into the human heart — his own! Despite the fact that his chief had forbidden the experiment, Forssmann went ahead and with the unsuspecting assistance of a nurse — Gerda Ditzen — cut down on his own left antecubital vein and inserted a ureteric catheter, which he advanced to his right atrium.

For the time being Forssmann disappears from the scene — he was not, presumably, very popular with his chief and met with much opposition — but others, Klein in Czechoslovakia (1930), Cournand and associates in the USA (1941), and McMichael and Sharpey-Schafer (1944) in England repeated the experiment. These workers were catheterising the right side of the heart in order to study the physiology of the cardiovascular system — they obtained blood samples to calculate cardiac output by the 'Fick' principle — but in 1944 Warren and his colleagues in the USA were the first to use cardiac catheterisation as a diagnostic technique. Their patient was a 44-year old man with an atrial septal defect, and Warren and his associates showed how the diagnosis could be confirmed by sampling blood of high oxygen saturation from the right atrium — the bright red colour of the samples was obvious to the naked eye.

So far catheterisation had been confined to the right side of the heart — though Warren had crossed the atrial septal defect (ASD) and placed the catheter in what he assumed, no doubt correctly, to be a pulmonary vein. Then, in 1950, Zimmerman, after some initial experiments on dogs, first catheterised the left side of the heart in man. He cut down on the artery in the antecubital fossa of a patient with aortic regurgitation and passed a catheter retrogradely through the aortic valve and into the left ventricle. The procedure was uncomplicated (apart from a few ventricular ectopic beats) but took 2 hours to complete. Today, when such procedures are routine and take but a few minutes, it is worth remembering how much courage and anxiety must have been involved in the first pioneering steps.

Although left heart catheterisation is now a routine procedure there are still occasions when entry to the left ventricle is difficult or impossible and the left atrium remains the most inaccessible of the cardiac chambers. Many techniques have been used to gain entry to the left atrium; few survive and several seem alarming to modern eyes. In France, Facquet (1952) described how it was possible to puncture the left atrium by a needle inserted through a bronchoscope ('transbronchial left heart catheterisation'), while in Sweden, Bjork (1953) approached the left heart by posterior transthoracic puncture. Radner (1954) employed suprasternal needle puncture — the needle passed in turn through the aorta and then the pulmonary artery before entering the left atrium. Only the transseptal technique first used on patients by Ross (1959) has survived the test of time and direct transthoracic needle puncture of the left ventricle (Brock) is occasionally employed today.

Percutaneous entry to the femoral artery was pioneered by Seldinger (1953) and modifications of his basic technique are probably the most widely used technique of vessel entry (artery or vein) in use in catheterisation laboratories today.

The history of angiography begins with non-selective (peripheral vein) injections, but in 1947 Chavez was the first to inject contrast medium directly into the heart via a cardiac catheter — *selective* angiography. In the 1950s many investigators attempted to visualise the coronary arteries angiographically. All these attempts were non-selective — contrast medium was injected into the aortic root and opacification of the coronary arteries was poor. Attempts to improve coronary opacification included inducing (temporary!) cardiac arrest with acetylcholine (Arnulf, 1958), and stopping antegrade aortic flow by occluding the aorta with a balloon (Dotter, 1958). It was left to Sones (1959) to develop the technique of *selective* injection of contrast medium into the coronary arteries. The first selective coronary arteriogram performed by Sones occurred by mistake — a powered injection of 30 cm^3 of contrast medium into the right coronary artery. Not surprisingly the patient became asystolic; Sones appreciated that a powerful cough will raise aortic pressure and improve coronary flow and the patient was still conscious enough to cooperate and survived without sequelae.

Sones used a brachial arteriotomy — this approach is often referred to as the 'Sones technique' as a result — but in 1962 Ricketts and Abrams employed a percutaneous transfemoral approach, and Judkins (1967) used the same approach and preshaped catheters to popularise what is probably the most commonly used technique of coronary arteriography today and is referred to as the 'Judkins technique'.

Many other developments are responsible for the safe and accurate nature of cardiac catheterisation; in particular the development of high-resolution X-ray imaging systems, which provide superb visualisation of fine intracardiac structures (angioplasty guide-wires have a 0.014" diameter) with very low levels of radiation. Nor should we forget that neither external cardiac massage nor direct current defibrillators were available to early workers — safety measures that may seldom be needed but which allow correction of what might otherwise be a disastrous complication.

The latest landmark in the development of cardiac catheterisation has been the introduction of *therapeutic* techniques; no longer is catheterisation merely a diagnostic technique, in many instances definitive treatment can be provided in the catheterisation laboratory. Cardiac pacing is the earliest example, and more recently catheter ablation of pathways leading to life-threatening arrhythmias has been shown to be possible. The use of catheter-mounted balloons was pioneered by Dotter and in 1964 Dotter and Judkins used a catheter to dilate stenoses in the arteries of the leg. It was Gruentzig who, in 1977, first used a catheter-mounted balloon to dilate a coronary artery stenosis — percutaneous transluminal coronary angioplasty (PTCA). The patient had a tight stenosis in the proximal left anterior descending coronary artery — he remains well and without evidence of ischaemia. But credit for the first therapeutic use of a balloon in the heart goes to Rashkind (1966) who transformed the outlook of infants with transposition of the great arteries by showing that it was possible to improve the mixing of pulmonary and systemic venous blood by tearing the atrial septum with a balloon mounted on the end of a catheter. Then, in 1982, Kan described the technique of balloon pulmonary valvuloplasty; the technique has re-placed surgical valvotomy for pulmonary stenosis and has led to similar methods of treatment for other stenosed valves and for coarctation.

Many other landmarks could be described; a patent ductus can be closed by a transcatheter technique and pathological vessels and fistulae can be closed by embolisation. What is certain is that developments will continue — almost certainly at an increasing pace — and that this short history will have to be rewritten to record future landmarks in the continuing development of cardiac catheterisation.

1 The 'tools' of catheterisation — cardiac catheters and how they are introduced and manipulated within the heart

Cardiac catheters

Catheters are so-called since Forssmann performed the first cardiac catheterisation in 1929 using a ureteric catheter. Originally catheters were simple tubes with a single end-hole; the 'Cournand' catheter is of this type. Today catheters come in a confusing variety of types, each designed for a specific purpose. A classification which will help to explain why a particular catheter is selected would recognise three main groups of cardiac catheters:

1 'Exploring' catheters.
2 Angiographic catheters.
3 'Interventional' catheters.

Exploring catheters. These are used for obtaining haemo-dynamic data: pressure measurements and blood samples from within the heart and great arteries. They have a single end-hole (for obtaining 'pulmonary capillary wedge pressure') though one, very useful, catheter (Goodale−Lubin) has two additional 'bird's eye' side-holes near the tip and others have two or more lumens and distal side-holes for recording simultaneous pressures from two sites ('double-lumen catheters'). Multiple side-holes, as in many 'Angiographic catheters', are a disadvantage in exploring the heart: a 'wedge' pressure cannot be obtained and false estimates of pressure gradients may result when some side-holes are in one chamber and the others in another. Exploring catheters may be of conventional type or may incorporate a balloon at the tip. The balloon is inflated with air (to avoid the danger of air embolism should the balloon rupture carbon dioxide must be used instead of air if there is a right-to-left shunt or if the catheter is used on the left side of the heart). When inflated the balloon carries the catheter with the blood stream; such balloon-tipped catheters (e.g. Swan−Ganz) are termed 'flow-guided' and are often used in catheterising infants and children with congenital heart disease. Flow-guided catheters may allow access to a site that cannot be reached with a conventional catheter and may help to obtain a 'wedge pressure' which is otherwise

1

unobtainable. Another advantage of these catheters is that the balloon spreads the force exerted on the myocardium so that they are safer and more 'gentle' than are conventional catheters.

One type of flow-guided, balloon-tipped, catheter incorporates a thermistor bead for the measurement of cardiac output by the thermodilution technique.

Angiographic catheters. A high-pressure jet of contrast medium emerging from the single end-hole of an exploring catheter would cause the catheter to recoil violently. Thus most angiographic catheters have multiple, opposed, side-holes through which the contrast medium can emerge. Some have a closed end (e.g. NIH, Eppendorf) but most have a fine end-hole to allow the use of a guide-wire. Angiographic catheters are of two main types; general purpose catheters used for ventriculography, aortography and pulmonary arteriography (e.g. NIH, Eppendorf, 'pigtail', Gensini) and special purpose, often preshaped, catheters such as are used for coronary arteriography (Judkins, Castillo, Amplatz). Angiographic versions of balloon-tipped, flow-guided, catheters are available. Some of the different types of cardiac catheters are illustrated in Fig. 1.1.

Interventional catheters. These catheters are used for *treating* cardiac lesions. Almost all incorporate a balloon of some sort. The most common interventional technique is 'percutaneous transluminal coronary angioplasty' (PTCA) and a wide variety of PTCA catheter systems are available. The first commonly used interventional technique was atrial septostomy (creating an atrial septal defect in neonates with complete transposition) developed by Rashkind — hence 'Rashkind septostomy catheter'. Other interventional techniques include pulmonary, aortic and mitral valvuloplasty, embolisation of unwanted vessels and angioplasty for 'recoarctation'. Suitable catheter systems are available for these and other interventional techniques. The use of these interventional catheters is described in Chapter 7.

Other important features in the choice of catheter include:
1 The material used in construction.
2 The external diameter of the shaft measured by the French gauge (F).

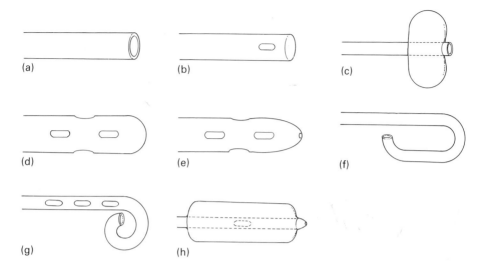

Fig. 1.1 Types of cardiac catheters. (a) Cournand, (b) Goodale–Lubin, and (c) Swan–Ganz monitoring are 'exploring' catheters; (d) NIH or Eppendorf, and (e) Gensini are general purpose angiographic catheters; (f) Left Judkins is an example of a preshaped catheter for coronary arteriography; (g) the pigtail is a very useful ventriculography catheter; and (h) is an example of an 'interventional' valvuloplasty catheter.

3 The maximum guide-wire diameter accepted by the end-hole.

4 The lumen diameter ('thin-wall' or standard) and the presence or absence of a wire mesh within the wall to improve torque control.

The external diameter of a catheter (its 'French gauge') can be divided by 3 to give the diameter in mm; thus a 6F catheter is 2 mm in diameter. Numbers 5–9F are commonly used.

Other 'tools' used in cardiac catheterisation

These include introducers, guide-wires, transseptal needle, sheaths and bioptomes.

Introducers. Cardiac catheterisation is often performed using a percutaneous approach to the vein or artery. Originally this was achieved by first puncturing the vessel with a needle through which a guide-wire could be passed into the vessel lumen. The needle was then removed and a tapered-tip catheter passed over the guide-wire and forced through the skin and subcutaneous tissues until it too lay within the vessel and the guide-wire could be removed (the Seldinger technique). Today it is more usual to employ a sheath introducer; the technique is much the same but a short, stiff, 'dilator' is used to form a track into the vessel and this dilator is housed within a short thin sheath. When the dilator is removed the sheath remains within the vessel allowing catheters to be inserted and changed without the need for a guide-wire; closed-end catheters can also be inserted through the sheath. Sheaths for arterial entry incorporate a one-way 'haemostatic valve' to prevent blood loss. The technique of percutaneous vessel entry using a sheath is illustrated in Fig. 1.2.

Introducing sheaths are usually short but long ones are available for special purposes; for example a 'long sheath' allows one to introduce a 'bioptome' into the left ventricle for 'endomyocardial biopsy'.

Guide-wires are constructed of a fine coiled wire around a central 'safety' core. They have a flexible tip which can be

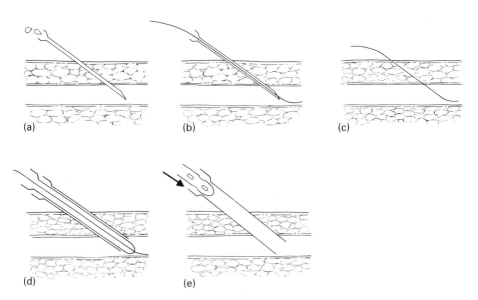

Fig. 1.2 Percutaneous entry to a vessel using a dilator and sheath. (a) The vessel is punctured using a short-bevel needle (bevel upwards). (b) Guide-wire with flexible tip introduced through the needle and into the vessel (artery or vein). (c) Needle removed leaving the guide-wire in place. (d) Dilator and sheath advanced over the guide-wire. (e) Dilator removed leaving the sheath in place ready to accept the cardiac catheter.

J-shaped and are usually Teflon coated for smoothness and to minimise thrombus formation. Guide-wires are used to lead a catheter through tortuous vessels or to assist in reaching a difficult position. Guide-wires are an essential component of coronary angioplasty systems.

Occasionally it is necessary to catheterise the left atrium by the 'transseptal' technique. A long needle is sheathed within a catheter and advanced from the femoral vein to the right atrium. When the correct position on the atrial septum is engaged by the catheter tip the needle is advanced (unsheathed) so as to puncture the interatrial septum. The catheter (or a dilator with a long sheath) is now advanced over the needle until it is free within the left atrium. The needle is then withdrawn and catheterisation proceeds. The transseptal technique is illustrated in Fig. 1.3.

Access to the heart

A catheterisation procedure is often referred to as a 'right heart' or a 'left heart' study (or both). By a right heart study we mean that the catheter is introduced through a vein from whence it can be advanced, via the superior or inferior vena cava, to the right atrium, the right ventricle and the pulmonary artery. A left heart study involves introducing the catheter into an artery and advancing it, against the

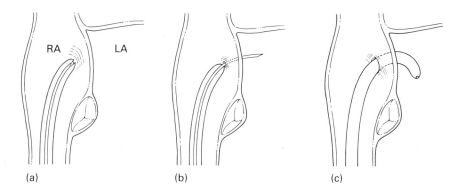

(a)   (b)   (c)

Fig. 1.3 The transseptal technique. (a) The catheter, with the long curved needle safely sheathed within it, is engaged against the limbus of the (closed) foramen ovale in the interatrial septum. (b) The needle is advanced (unsheathed) so as to puncture the atrial septum. If left atrial pressure is then recorded it is safe to advance the catheter over the needle so as to enter the left atrium, (c) when the needle can be withdrawn.

direction of the blood flow, until it enters the aorta and can cross the aortic valve (when that valve is open) to enter the left ventricle. In patients with congenital heart disease the distinction often becomes blurred as intracardiac defects may allow the catheter, though introduced through a vein, to enter the left side of the heart from the right side. Thus we have a number of possible sites of entry — some are veins and others are arteries. Arteries and veins lie side-by-side so that an anatomical site such as the antecubital fossa (at the elbow) or the inguinal region (the groin) allows entry to both an artery and a vein. The first choice that the operator has to make is whether to approach from the arm or from the leg. The choice is influenced by the object of the study but also by the chosen technique; in general vessels in the groin (femoral artery and vein) are entered *percutaneously* and those at the elbow by a *cut-down*.

The antecubital fossa. This 'from the arm' approach to the brachial vein and artery provides easy access to the right ventricle, pulmonary artery and wedge position when a vein is cannulated. When the brachial artery is cannulated the approach affords a higher chance of crossing a stenotic aortic valve than when the approach is from the leg. A cut-down is the usual technique. After the injection of a local anaesthetic (e.g. 1% lidocaine) a short transverse incision is made in the skin and the vessels exposed by blunt dissection while an assistant retracts the skin and subcutaneous tissues. Ligatures are passed around the vein and tapes around the artery to provide haemostasis and a small incision in the artery or vein allows the catheter to be introduced. At the end of the procedure the vessels are repaired. Repairing an arteriotomy requires meticulous technique; the major complication to be feared is loss of the radial pulse following a poor repair though this complication should occur in less than 0.5% of cases. The technique of arterial cut-down is illustrated in Fig. 1.4. The advantage of an arteriotomy is that the patient can be allowed home the same day and studies can be on a 'day case' basis.

The inguinal approach. This approach to the femoral vein and artery is usually performed percutaneously using an introducing sheath as described earlier and illustrated in

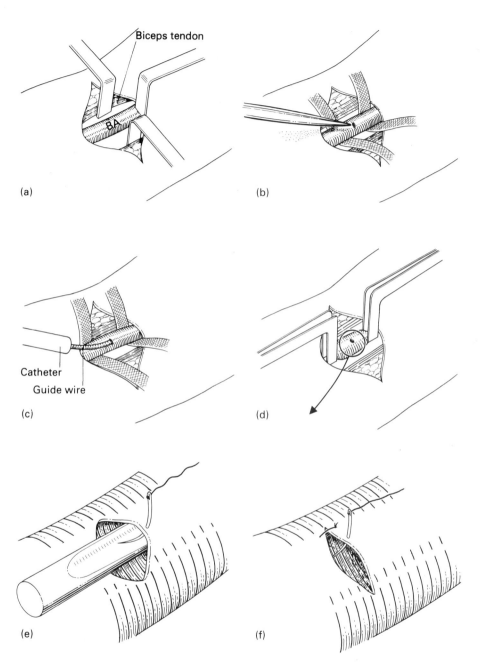

(a) Exposure of the brachial artery (BA) by retracting the biceps tendon laterally. (b) Incision in the artery. Tapes are around the artery to control bleeding. (c) Guide wire introduced; the catheter will be advanced over the guide wire. (d) Arterial repair. Haemostasis obtained by using angled arterial clamps. (e) Using an upside-down introducer to guard the posterior arterial wall during insertion of the first sutures. (f) The repair in progress using interrupted 6/o sutures.

Fig. 1.2. Once the sheath(s) are in position catheterisation can proceed rapidly and multiple catheter changes can be made through the ready access provided by the sheaths. The approach to the right heart from the femoral vein provides the best chance of entering the left atrium (and thence the left heart) via a 'patent foramen ovale' or an atrial septal defect. For this reason the approach is the favoured one for most cases of congenital heart disease. Some procedures can only, or can best, be performed by this approach, examples include atrial septostomy, pulmonary and aortic valvuloplasty, coronary angioplasty and coarctation angioplasty.

There are other possible sites of access. In neonates the umbilical artery and vein are occasionally used as is a cutdown on the axillary artery and vein. The subclavian vein is often entered percutaneously and is a favoured approach for pacemaker wire insertion.

Manipulation of the catheter within the heart

To the layperson, watching catheterisation for the first time, it seems amazing that the catheter can be manipulated so easily to any position within the heart and great vessels. The secret is simple: most catheters have a curve moulded a few centimetres from the tip. Because of this curve simple rotational movement of the catheter shaft results in changes in the direction in which the tip is pointing. In addition advancing the catheter may cause the tip to impinge against the wall of the heart or vessel so that further advance causes a 'loop' to form. All catheter manipulation is achieved by rotation and advance or retraction of the shaft of the catheter. Of course all such manipulation is done under fluoroscopic control. In addition the waveform obtained is constantly displayed and together these items of information — the fluoroscopic display and the pressure record — tell the operator where the tip of the catheter is lying. In doubtful cases the operator may make use of small 'scout injections' of contrast medium. Biplane fluoroscopy may be used (if available) or may be rotated the X-ray tube and intensifier so as to be able to distinguish between anterior and posterior positions of the catheter tip. Difficult manipulations may be helped by the use of a guide-wire or a balloon-tipped catheter. The steps involved in manipulating a catheter from the superior vena cava through the

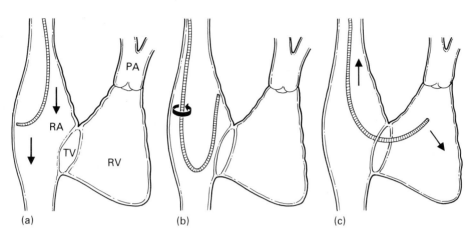

Fig. 1.5 Entering the right ventricle (and pulmonary artery) from the right atrium, (a) abut the catheter against lateral wall of right atrium to form a loop; (b) rotate the loop so that the loop is directed medially with the catheter tip against the interatrial septum; (c) withdraw the catheter so that the tip travels down the atrial septum and then 'flips' through the tricuspid valve pointing towards the right ventricular outflow tract.

right atrium and ventricle to the pulmonary artery are illustrated in Fig. 1.5.

One site reached by right heart catheterisation needs some explanation. This is the 'wedge' or 'pulmonary capillary wedge' position. This is obtained when a catheter is advanced so far out into the pulmonary arterial tree that it blocks the vessel that it is in. At this point all flow ceases in the segment of the pulmonary vasculature beyond the occluding catheter and the catheter (which must have an end-hole) now records the left atrial pressure — or something very close to it. This is fortunate since the left atrium is the one chamber that cannot easily be reached by either right or left heart catheterisation.

2 How data obtained during catheterisation are used to make the diagnosis

Although many specialised techniques have been used in the catheterisation laboratory, three techniques form the basis of nearly all diagnostic procedures. These are: (1) the measurement of *pressure* within the heart and great vessels; (2) the measurement of *oxygen saturation* of samples of blood withdrawn from sites within the heart and great vessels; and (3) *angiography*.

The measurement of pressure

A cardiac catheter is a hollow tube which is filled with liquid (saline, dextrose solution). Thus a pressure generated within the cardiac chamber in which the open tip of the catheter is positioned, will be transmitted to the hub of the catheter by the column of fluid within the catheter. The hub of the catheter is attached to a *pressure transducer*. A transducer is simply a device that transforms one form of energy into another; in this case mechanical energy (pressure) into electrical energy. The fluid within the catheter and the 'dome' of the transducer is in contact with a stiff metal diaphragm and the pressure waves displace this diaphragm (by a very small amount). The movement of the diaphragm is arranged to stretch two wires of a 'Wheatstone bridge' (or a silicon crystal with similar configuration), thus altering their resistance and causing a small electrical current to flow. This current is amplified and the resulting signal may then be displayed on an oscilloscope and used to drive some form of strip-chart recorder (Fig. 2.1).

The technician responsible for recording has a very important part to play. First of all the transducer, pressure line(s) and taps must be connected to a pressurised bag of heparinised saline (or dextrose, Hartmann's solution, etc.) and the system flushed through. It is important that there are no air bubbles in the system (and that there is fluid behind the dome of a disposable transducer). Air bubbles are a major cause of 'damping' — the system will not respond to rapid changes in pressure and the record will underestimate the true pressure as well as blurring the waveform. The transducer has then to be adjusted to the

10

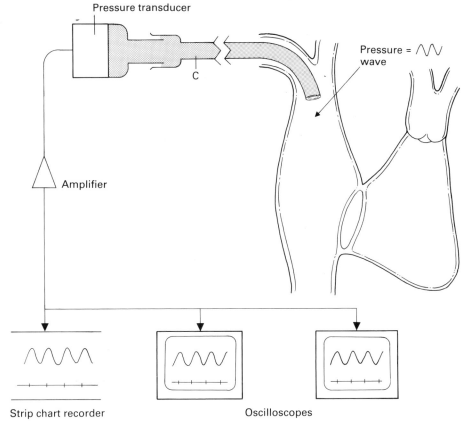

Pressure transducer

Pressure = /\/\/
wave

Amplifier

C

Strip chart recorder

Oscilloscopes

Fig. 2.1 Recording and displaying intracardiac pressures. The pressure waves within the heart are transmitted through the hollow fluid-filled catheter (C) to the pressure transducer, which transforms the mechanical pressure into an electrical signal. This electrical signal is amplified and then recorded on a strip-chart recorder and displayed on oscilloscopes in front of the operator and the recording technician.

same level as the middle of the patient's chest ('mid-chest' is the conventional zero reference point for cardiac catheterisation). Finally the system has to be calibrated by opening the transducer dome to atmospheric pressure (mid-chest and zero) and to a column of fluid of known height providing a known pressure in mmHg. The amplifiers have to be balanced with the zero and calibration pressures set to the desired level on the oscilloscope at several alternative sensitivities.

Pressure records provide diagnostic information in three ways:

1 We may study the *waveform*.

2 We obtain information from the *absolute value* of the pressures recorded.

3 We can *compare* two (or more) pressures, which can be recorded simultaneously and the records superimposed on the strip chart.

Waveform

Three distinct waveforms can be obtained from within the heart and great vessels. These are (i) atrial, (ii) ventricular, and (iii) arterial waveforms.

Atrial pressure waves (Fig. 2.2). These are obtained from the right and left atria and from the systemic and pulmonary veins that connect to them. Atrial pressures are usually of low amplitude (around 5 mmHg, in the right atrium and 10 mmHg in the left atrium). In the normal heart (in sinus rhythm) there are two positive and two negative waves in each cardiac cycle. The 'a' wave is due to atrial systole (contraction) and its onset coincides with the 'p' wave of the electrocardiogram, which signals atrial contraction. The 'a' wave is followed by the 'x' descent (as the atrium relaxes) and then a second positive deflection; the 'v' wave. The 'v' wave coincides with ventricular systole as the atrium fills while the exit (tricuspid or mitral) valve is closed and coincides with the 'T' wave on the electrocardiogram. The 'v' wave is followed by the 'y' descent as the atrium empties passively during ventricular diastole (relaxation).

Ventricular pressure waves (Fig. 2.3(a)). These have a roughly rectangular shape. There is a steep upward deflection as pressure rises during systole before the exit (pulmonary and aortic) valves have opened ('isometric contraction') followed by a more-or-less rounded peak during ejection. There follows a steep vertical decline ('isometric relaxation'), *which reaches near-zero pressure*. During ventricular diastole, filling of the ventricle causes a gradual rise in pressure with a terminal 'hump' due to atrial contraction ('a' wave) before once again the pressure rises steeply as the ventricle contracts with the next cardiac cycle (signalled by the 'QRS' complex of the electrocardiogram).

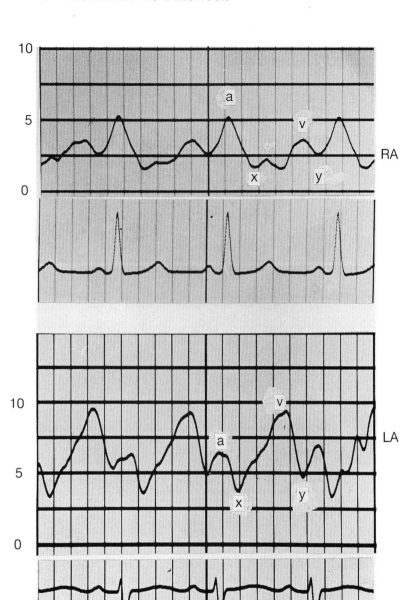

Fig. 2.2 Atrial pressure waveform. Normal right (upper panel) and left (lower panel) atrial pressure tracings. The 'a' wave is dominant in the right atrium and the 'v' wave in the left atrium. There are two positive deflections (waves) in each cardiac cycle. The pressure is of low amplitude — less than 10 mmHg.

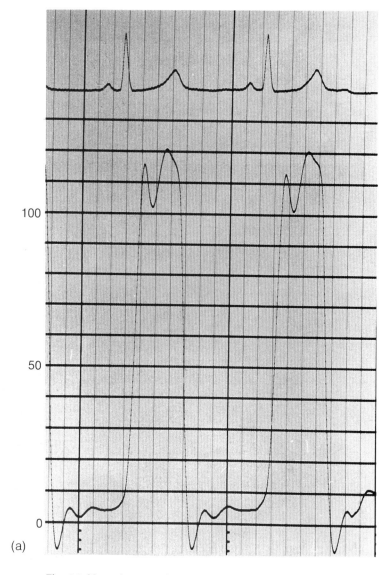

100

50

0

(a)

Fig. 2.3 Normal ventricular (a) and arterial (b) waveforms. Note how the recording technician has increased the electronic damping at the end of the arterial recording to obtain a *mean* arterial pressure.

Arterial pressure waves (Fig. 2.3(b)). These have a more-or-less triangular form. Pressure rises with the onset of ejection and then declines more slowly to the diastolic pressure until interrupted by the next ejection. This decline is often interrupted by a small notch (the dicrotic notch), which

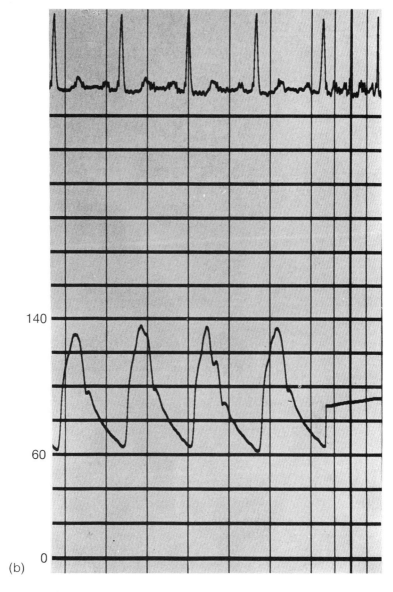

Fig. 2.3 *continued.*

occurs as the outlet (semilunar — aortic or pulmonary) valves close. Unlike a ventricular pressure, arterial pressure waves *do not decline to zero*. The normal pulmonary diastolic pressure is around 10–15 mmHg and aortic diastolic pressure around 80–90 mmHg.

Waveform helps the operator in two ways. Most importantly, it indicates where the catheter tip is lying — in an atrium, a ventricle or a great artery. This information cannot always be deduced by inspection of the fluoroscopic display. Secondly there may be abnormalities of waveform which suggest a diagnosis. For example, severe tricuspid or mitral regurgitation result in the production of a large 'v' wave so that atrial pressure comes to resemble ventricular pressure (ventricularisation). But abnormalities of waveform by themselves are seldom enough to provide a certain diagnosis. Abnormalities of waveform associated with certain conditions will be discussed in the appropriate sections on congenital and acquired heart disease.

Absolute pressure

Pressures within the heart are measured in millimetres of mercury (mmHg). The normal right ventricular systolic pressure does not exceed 25–30 mmHg. Thus if a catheter is within the right ventricle and recording a (ventricular) systolic pressure of for example 90 mmHg, there is clearly some cardiac abnormality and the cause of this high right ventricular pressure must be sought. The possibilities include outflow obstruction (infundibular or pulmonary valve stenosis), pulmonary vascular disease, a high downstream (pulmonary vein) pressure or a communication between the right and left heart (e.g. a ventricular septal defect — VSD). By itself, therefore, the absolute level of pressure seldom provides a complete diagnosis. Further information must be obtained, and this is often provided by comparing one pressure with another — comparative pressures. A table of normal intracardiac pressures will be found in Chapter 9.

*Comparative
pressures*

In the example given above a high right ventricular pressure suggested four possibilities: outflow obstruction, pulmonary vascular disease, a high pulmonary vein pressure or an intracardiac communication. If in the same patient the catheter is now advanced to enter the pulmonary artery and the systolic pressure here is found to be, say, 10 mmHg, then outflow tract obstruction (e.g. pulmonary stenosis) is established as the cause of the high right ventricular pressure. Pressure has fallen beyond the site of obstruction. The

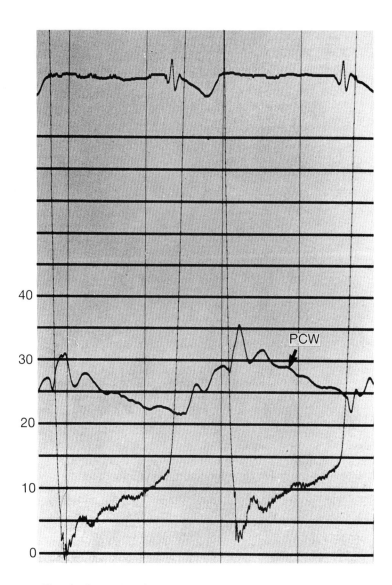

Fig. 2.4 Comparison between two simultaneously recorded pressures providing diagnostic information. (a) *Mitral stenosis*. There is a pressure gradient between the wedge pressure (p.c.w.) and the diastolic pressure in the left ventricle. Normally both pressures will have equalised by mid-diastole. Both pressures are recorded at the same high level of amplification ('range'), so that the systolic portion of the left ventricular pressure wave is off the top of the chart; (*continues opposite*).

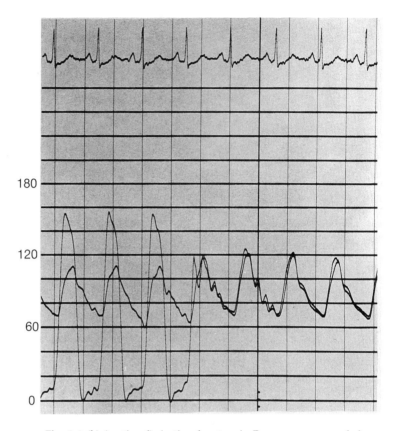

Fig. 2.4 (b) (*continued*) *Aortic valve stenosis*. Pressures are recorded, simultaneously and at the same amplification, from the aorta and from the left ventricle and show a pressure gradient. The left ventricular catheter is withdrawn to the aorta half-way through the record and there is an abrupt change to an arterial pressure wave showing that the obstruction was at the level of the arterial (aortic) valve.

difference between the two pressures is referred to as the pressure *gradient*.

If, however, pulmonary arterial systolic pressure is found to be the same as right ventricular systolic pressure, another cause must be sought. If right ventricular pressure is identical to left ventricular pressure then a VSD is a likely diagnosis, as a large VSD allows equalisation of pressures between the two ventricles; further information, including angiography, will be needed to confirm the diagnosis. The elucidation of the causes of 'pulmonary hypertension' will be discussed later.

Important examples of the comparison between two pressures include the investigation of stenotic valves. In mitral stenosis there will be a pressure gradient between the left atrium and left ventricle during diastole. In aortic stenosis there will be a gradient between the left ventricle and the aorta during systole (Fig. 2.4). The magnitude of the gradient is a guide to the severity of stenosis.

The measurement of oxygen saturation

In the catheterisation laboratory the oxygen saturation of blood samples withdrawn from the heart is measured by 'reflection oximetry'. When blood is fully saturated with oxygen it is bright red in colour; when the oxygen saturation is low the blood (haemoglobin) is purple. The higher the oxygen saturation the redder is the sample. This is made use of in reflection oximetry. A small sample of blood (as little as 0.4 ml in some oximeters) is placed in the oximeter where light shining on the sample is reflected on to a photo-cell (through suitable filters) and the resulting current is proportional to the redness of the sample. Reflection oximetry allows the percentage saturation to be read directly to an accuracy of one or two percentage points and within 15–20 s.

Measurements of oxygen saturation provide diagnostic information in two ways:
1 By comparing the saturations of samples taken from a number of sites we can detect the presence of an intracardiac 'shunt' and can localise that shunt as occurring at atrial, ventricular or arterial level. The following example should serve to illustrate this diagnostic use of measurements of oxygen saturation.

A series of samples are taken with the following values of oxygen saturation:

Sample from:	Oxygen saturation
Pulmonary artery	87%
Right ventricle	88%
Right atrium	70%
Superior vena cava	68%
Inferior vena cava	72%

It is clear that there is an increase in oxygen saturation occurring in the right ventricle — in the jargon there is a left-to-right shunt, or 'step-up', at ventricular level and a VSD is one possible diagnosis.

2   The second, and very important, diagnostic use of oxygen saturation measurements is in the calculation of cardiac output and related measurements by the *Fick* method. The method is best illustrated by a simple analogy (Fig. 2.5). Imagine a stream of shoppers entering a store. Each is observed to be carrying (say) one loaf of bread on entering the store. As they leave it is observed that each is now carrying two loaves — each has added one loaf to his shopping basket. If we know how many loaves of bread were sold in a given time (1 min) we can calculate how many shoppers passed through the store in that time. In this analogy the loaves of bread represent *units of oxygen*. Each shopper represents a *unit of blood*. The store represents the lungs. Thus if we calculate (from measurement of oxygen saturation) that the oxygen content of pulmonary arterial blood entering the lungs is 180 ml/l and of pulmonary venous blood leaving the lungs is 200 ml/l, then 20 ml of oxygen/l are added to the blood as it passes through the lungs. If we measure the amount of oxygen taken up by the lungs in 1 min (the 'oxygen consumption') and find it to be 100 ml, it is clear that 5l of blood must have passed through the lungs during that minute (100/20 = 5). In the normal heart the volume of blood passing through the lungs is the same as that passing through the body (since the two circulations are 'in series') and we have thus measured the *cardiac output*. Details of the calculation (somewhat simplified here) will be found in Chapter 9. In a patient with congenital heart disease and with an intra-cardiac shunt, the volumes of blood flowing through the pulmonary and systemic circulation are *not* the same; with a pure left-to-right shunt, pulmonary flow will be greater than systemic flow, when the shunt is from right-to-left the reverse is true. However, we can measure pulmonary and systemic flow separately. Pulmonary flow was given by the oxygen consumption divided by the *pulmonary* arteriovenous (AV) oxygen difference (pulmonary vein oxygen content minus pulmonary artery oxygen content). Similarly systemic flow can be calculated as the oxygen consumption divided by the *systemic* AV oxygen difference (systemic arterial oxygen content minus 'mixed systemic venous' oxygen

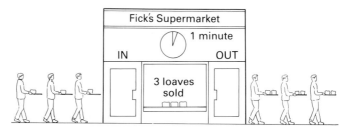

Fig. 2.5 The Fick principle. If three loaves of bread are sold in 1 min and each customer added one loaf to his shopping basket then three customers must have passed through the supermarket during that 1 min.

content). The difference between systemic and pulmonary flow is a measure of the size of the shunt.

The calculations of systemic and pulmonary flow and of shunt size are not performed until after the study is completed. However, the operator can obtain a rough idea of what the values will be during the study; since pulmonary flow is given by the oxygen consumption divided by the pulmonary AV oxygen difference and since pulmonary vein saturation is almost always about 97%, the major variable is the saturation of pulmonary arterial blood. If this value is high the AV difference will be small and pulmonary flow will turn out to be high — and vice versa. Similarly a low systemic flow will be present if the systemic AV difference is large, as may be suggested by a low mixed venous saturation. Finally a large step-up in the right side of the heart will imply a large left-to-right shunt, while severe arterial desaturation will imply a large right-to-left shunt.

Combining pressure and flow measurements — pulmonary resistance

An important reason for catheterising many patients (especially those with congenital heart disease) is to measure the pulmonary resistance. In electrical terms the resistance (R) of a circuit is given by:

$$R = V/I$$

(Ohm's law) where V (volts) is equivalent to *pressure* and I (amperes) to *flow*. We make use of exactly the same relationship in cardiology. Thus the 'resistance' to flow through a circulation can be expressed as the mean pressure in the artery supplying the circulation divided by the flow through the circulation. If mean pressure is expressed in mmHg and flow in l/min, the resistance is given in so-called 'Wood units' (after Paul Wood, cardiologist at the Brompton and National Heart Hospitals). The symbols are changed from those used in Ohm's law:

R (resistance) = P (mean pressure) / Q (flow)

Mean pressure is usually obtained electronically but, if only systolic and diastolic arterial pressures are available, a close approximation is given by:

$[(S - D)/3] + D$

where S = systolic pressure and D = diastolic pressure (this only works for an arterial pressure of triangular form; but it is arterial pressures that concern us).

The significance of measurements of resistance is most easily explained by considering 'pulmonary hypertension'. By pulmonary hypertension we simply mean that the pressure in the pulmonary artery is significantly higher than the normal (systolic) pressure of 25–30 mmHg. Pulmonary hypertension can arise in three ways:

1   The pressure in the pulmonary veins is abnormally high so that pulmonary arterial pressure has to rise to overcome this high 'downstream' pressure; mitral stenosis and left ventricular failure are examples of this mechanism.

2   There is a high resistance to flow through the vessels (usually the arterioles) of the pulmonary vascular bed because they have become narrowed or obstructed; pulmonary vascular disease and pulmonary embolism are examples of this mechanism.

3   There is a high flow through the pulmonary circulation; usually because of a communication with the systemic circulation as in a ventricular septal defect.

Note that of the three mechanisms that result in pulmonary hypertension only one is due to a high *resistance* or 'pulmonary vascular disease'.

The general formula for calculating 'resistance' as described above is:

$R = P/Q$

where R = resistance in Wood units, P = mean pressure in mmHg and Q = blood flow in l/min. To allow for the effect of downstream pressure we can modify this expression by subtracting left atrial (or wedge) pressure:

$$R_{pa} = (P_{pa} - P_{la})/Q_{pa}$$

where P_{pa} = mean pulmonary artery pressure in mmHg, P_{la} = mean left atrial (or wedge) pressure in mmHg, Q_{pa} = pulmonary artery blood flow in l/min, and R_{pa} = the resistance to flow due to the pulmonary vascular bed alone and is referred to as 'the pulmonary arteriolar resistance'.

Four examples will suffice to explain how resistance measurements provide diagnostic information and allow us to distinguish between the three possible mechanisms that lead to pulmonary hypertension. These examples are illustrated in Fig. 2.6.

1   In a person with a normal heart we measure a mean pulmonary artery pressure of 20 mmHg, a mean left atrial pressure of 10 mmHg and a pulmonary blood flow of 5 l/min. Substituting in the equation we obtain:

$$R_{pa} = 20 - 10/5 \quad = 2.0 \text{ units}$$

These are normal values.

2   In a patient with mitral stenosis the mean pulmonary artery pressure is raised at 30 mmHg, the mean left atrial pressure is raised at 20 mmHg and pulmonary flow is normal at 5 l/min. In this case the calculation is:

$$R_{pa} = 30 - 20/5 \quad = 2 \text{ units}$$

We have determined that pulmonary arteriolar resistance is normal — there is no pulmonary vascular disease — and that the raised pulmonary artery pressure is due to a high downstream (left atrial) pressure.

3   In a patient with 'primary pulmonary hypertension' mean pulmonary artery pressure is again raised at 30 mmHg, flow is again normal at 5 l/min and the left atrial mean pressure is normal at 10 mmHg:

$$R_{pa} = 30 - 10/5 \quad = 4 \text{ units}$$

and the cause of the pulmonary hypertension in this patient is an abnormally high pulmonary arteriolar resistance — pulmonary vascular disease.

4   Finally a patient with a ventricular septal defect has a

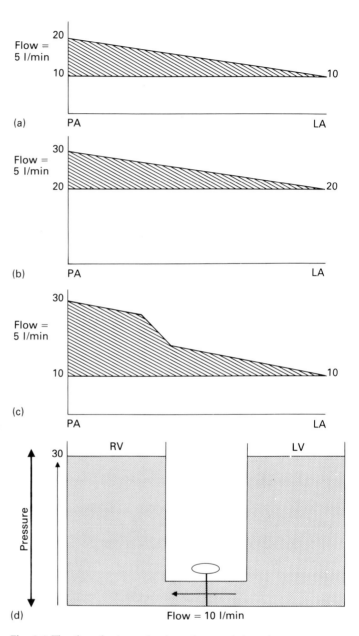

Fig. 2.6 The three basic mechanisms that result in pulmonary hypertension. (a) The normal situation. (b) High downstream pressure (e.g. mitral stenosis). (c) Raised pulmonary resistance (e.g. primary pulmonary hypertension. (d) High flow. The water level (pressure) in the left-hand drum (RV) will equalise with that in the right-hand drum (LV) as a result of flow from the high-pressure to the low-pressure chamber (from LV to RV).

raised mean pulmonary artery pressure of 30 mmHg, and a normal left atrial pressure of 10 mmHg. So far the findings are the same as in the previous patient with pulmonary vascular disease, but when the pulmonary blood flow is measured we find a narrow AV oxygen difference (high pulmonary artery saturation) and pulmonary flow is calculated and found to be increased at 10 l/min.

$$R_{pa} = 30 - 10/10 \quad = 2 \text{ units}$$

Pulmonary hypertension in this patient was simply due to the high flow — the left-to-right shunt — and there is no pulmonary vascular disease.

In some patients there may be more than one mechanism responsible for pulmonary hypertension; patients with mitral stenosis and a high left atrial pressure may develop secondary pulmonary vascular disease, as may patients with a left-to-right shunt, when the process is referred to as 'the Eisenmenger reaction'. But by measuring flow and pressure we can still determine the diagnosis and the relative contributions of each mechanism.

While the measurement of pressure poses no major problems the measurement of flow by the Fick method does. In particular, oxygen consumption is often taken from tables of normal values with a potential for serious error. When the accurate measurement of resistance is crucial, then oxygen consumption has to be measured or an alternative method (such as thermodilution) used to determine pulmonary flow.

Measurement of cardiac output by thermodilution

The blood flow (Q) through an organ, such as the lungs, can be calculated from the general formula:

$$Q = I/ct$$

Where I is the amount of an *indicator* injected into the vessel supplying the circulation and ct is the mean concentration of the indicator (c) in unit time (t) in the effluent blood. If a dye is used as the indicator and concentration in the effluent is plotted continuously a characteristic curve will be inscribed (Fig. 2.7).

The area under this curve is proportional to the mean concentration. Unfortunately some particles of dye will reappear (recirculate) before inscription of the primary curve

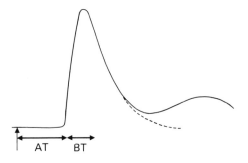

Fig. 2.7 A typical indicator dilution curve. The time at which indicator was injected is marked by an arrow. The time taken for the first particles of indicator to appear at the sampling site is the 'appearance time' (AT). The concentration of indicator at the sampling site increases for a time (the 'build-up time' — BT) to a peak concentration and then decays (the 'disappearance phase') until a secondary increase in concentration results from the reappearance of the fastest travelling particles of indicator at the sampling site. This reappearance phase interrupts the primary curve, which would otherwise decay exponentially as indicated by the dotted line.

is complete and this makes it difficult to measure the area under the primary curve in order to obtain ct. Thermodilution avoids this problem by using cold saline as the indicator. The saline is warmed by passage through the lungs and the primary curve is not distorted. In practice a catheter is used which has a thermistor bead at its tip. This detects the 'cold' as it arrives in the pulmonary artery and sends the signal to a computer, which calculates the area under the curve and thus the cardiac output. A number of readings are obtained and averaged. Thermodilution is a simple, and infinitely repeatable, method of obtaining a reasonably accurate measurement of cardiac output that is often used in both the catheterisation laboratory and the intensive care unit.

So far we have considered two of the three basic techniques used to obtain diagnostic information by cardiac catheterisation — the measurement of pressure and the measurement of oxygen saturation together with the calculated variables derived from these measurements. The third basic diagnostic technique — angiography — is so important that it is given a chapter to itself, Chapter 3.

3 The performance and interpretation of angiograms

Strictly, angiography refers to the injection of contrast medium into *vessels*; 'angiocardiography' refers to both intravascular and intracardiac injections, while other terms, such as 'aortography', 'ventriculography', etc., are self-explanatory. For simplicity, the term angiography will be used here to cover all investigations involving the injection of radio-opaque contrast medium into the heart or great vessels. The first 'angiograms' performed on patients with heart disease were 'non-selective'; contrast medium was injected into peripheral veins and opacified all the cardiac chambers in turn. Today we talk of 'selective angiography' since contrast medium is injected centrally and the site of injection selected according to the specific anomaly that is to be demonstrated.

Contrast media are opaque to X-rays by virtue of their iodine content; the amount of iodine present is indicated by a number, so that, for example, Isopaque 440 contains 440 mg iodine/ml and Omnipaque 350 contains 350 mg iodine/ml. In solution, conventional contrast media dissolve into anions and cations that possess a very high osmolality (1500–2000 mOsm/kg — the osmolality of blood is 300 mOsm/kg). While higher concentrations of iodine provide greater radio-opacity, it is unfortunate that higher concentrations also result in the medium being more viscous, with a higher osmolality in relation to blood. Most of the side-effects that follow angiography are due to the high osmolality; newer non-ionic media (such as Omnipaque — iohexol) have a lower osmolality than conventional media, such as Isopaque and Urograffin, and cause fewer side-effects. The headache that commonly follows angiography with conventional contrast media is less severe or even absent. Unfortunately the 'non-ionic' media are much more expensive and tend to be more viscous than conventional media. Viscosity is important as it limits our ability to inject a large volume of contrast medium, rapidly, through a long thin catheter. Viscosity is less at 37°C than at room temperature; for this reason all contrast media should be warmed before use.

The injection of contrast medium through a long thin catheter requires a powered injector pump that can generate a high pressure. Modern angiographic injectors can be programmed to inject a given quantity of contrast medium at a preset *rate*. A rough guide to the volume of contrast medium needed for adequate opacification of a cardiac chamber is 1 ml/kg body weight — less in adults and rather more in infants and children if the chamber to be opacified is large or 'volume loaded' because of a left-to-right shunt or valvar regurgitation.

In most cases filming is with 35-mm cine-film at speeds of 25 to 50 f.p.s. Some installations allow large-format limited-number (20—30) serial films to be taken at maximum rates of 4—6 f.p.s., and such films provide exquisite detail for purposes such as pulmonary arteriography. Cine-film is viewed on a special projector (e.g. Tagarno) that allows variable-speed viewing with instant stop, reverse or forward motion.

X-rays are generated within the X-ray tube when a beam of electrons from the cathode hits the tungsten anode. This generates considerable heat so that the anode is made to rotate thereby allowing only a small portion of the anode to be used at any one moment. Cine-film is more sensitive to light than to X-rays so that, having passed through the patient, the X-rays are made to impinge on the 'input phosphor' of an 'image intensifier' where the image is converted to a light image. The intensity of this light image is greatly increased (made brighter) within the image intensifier before passing through a collector lens system and 'image distributor', which splits the light beam between the cine- and TV cameras (Fig. 3.1).

Modern angiography equipment allows the operator to rotate the linked X-ray tube and image intensifier in two planes; the suspension can be rotated in the sagittal plane providing views anywhere between anteroposterior and lateral and, in addition, can be given variable degrees of cranial or caudal tilt. This facility is of great importance since the aim is to view a three-dimensional structure — the heart — in such a way that the area of interest is perpendicular to the X-ray beam and not foreshortened or obscured by overlapping structures. Some installations allow simultaneous filming in two planes — *biplane angiography*.

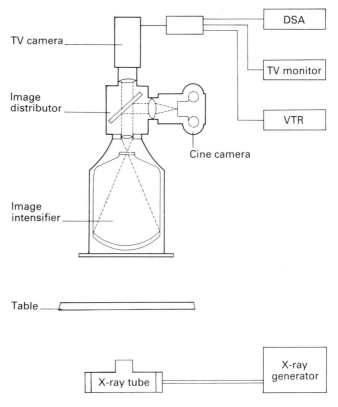

TV camera

Image
distributor

Image
intensifier

Table

X-ray tube

DSA

TV monitor

VTR

Cine camera

X-ray
generator

Fig. 3.1 Diagrammatic representation of X-ray apparatus used in cardiac catheterisation.

Biplane angiography has the advantage that two views are obtained using only a single injection of contrast medium. In infants and children the total amount of contrast medium that can safely be given is strictly limited (to a total of about 4 ml/kg), and for this reason biplane units are used in centres engaged in the study of congenital heart disease — paediatric cardiology units.

The interpretation of angiograms

It is not always appreciated that angiograms provide *physiological* as well as *anatomical* information. That the shape and position of a heart chamber or vessel is displayed by angiography is obvious, i.e. structural information is displayed. But angiography does much more; in particular, angiography provides information about the presence and severity of valvar regurgitation, about the volume of blood flow through a vessel or heart chamber, about ventricular function and about the presence and position of intracardiac shunts or abnormally connected vessels.

Valvar heart disease. This important subject will be discussed more fully in a later chapter (Chapter 6), but the principles of the angiographic study of valve disease can be outlined here. When a heart valve is diseased it may become narrowed ('stenosed') or it may leak (e.g. mitral 'regurgitation' or 'incompetence'). When a heart valve leaks some of the blood downstream will pass backwards; during ventricular systole at the atrioventricular (tricuspid and mitral) valves and during diastole at the ventriculoarterial (aortic and pulmonary) valves. If this downstream blood is opacified by the injection of contrast medium into the downstream chamber or vessel then the contrast medium will be seen to opacify the upstream chamber. The rapidity and density of opacification can be used as a guide to the severity of regurgitation, (Fig. 3.2).

A leaking valve imposes *a volume load* on the ventricle, which has to pump the normal forward flow *plus* the extra volume of blood that has leaked backwards. This results in a proportional increase in the size of the ventricle, which provides a second index of the severity of regurgitation. This relationship between the size of a heart chamber or vessel is the basis of the second way in which angiography provides *physiological* information.

The relationship between blood flow and chamber or vessel size. There is a roughly linear relationship between the volume of blood flowing through a vessel or heart chamber and the size (diameter, volume) of the vessel or chamber. This can most easily be understood if we take some examples of abnormalities that alter the normal flow through a vessel. We tend to think of the aorta as being a large vessel and the brachial artery a small one 'because they were made that way'. But in 'aortic atresia' — a congenital cardiac anomaly in which the only blood flow through the ascending aorta is that supplying the coronary circulation — this vessel is a minute structure (Fig. 3.3.1b). Conversely a patient with an arteriovenous fistula in the forearm will have an enormously dilated brachial artery reflecting the torrential blood flow through the fistula.

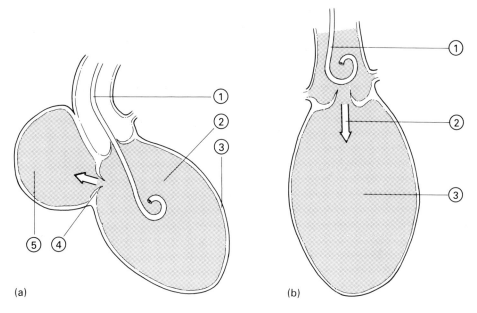

(a)

(b)

Fig. 3.2 The angiographic diagnosis of valvar regurgitation. (a) *Mitral regurgitation* — right oblique projection. (1) Catheter passed into left ventricle from aorta. (2) Contrast medium injected into left ventricle. (3) The left ventricle is enlarged to accommodate the increased volume of blood due to regurgitant flow. (4) Contrast medium passes 'backwards' through the leaking mitral valve. (5) The left atrium is opacified as a result of regurgitation. The degree and rapidity of opacification of the left atrium is a guide to the severity of mitral regurgitation. (b) *Aortic regurgitation* — left oblique projection. (1) Contrast medium injected into the aorta above the aortic valve. (2) Contrast medium passes into the left ventricle through the leaking aortic valve. (3) The degree and rapidity of opacification of the ventricle is a guide to the severity of aortic regurgitation.

This relationship between vessel size and blood flow is of most practical use in determining pulmonary blood flow. In conditions with a low blood flow to the pulmonary arteries — such as the tetralogy of Fallot or pulmonary atresia — the pulmonary arteries are very small (Fig. 3.3.2b). Indeed they may be so small that surgical correction is impossible until they have been caused to enlarge by increasing the blood flow through them by inserting a surgical ('Blalock') shunt. Conversely, the pulmonary arteries are very large when, as in atrial septal defect, there is a large left-to-right shunt and a high pulmonary flow (Fig. 3.3.3). Unfortunately the pulmonary arteries tend to remain dilated even after the flow has been reduced (after surgical cor-

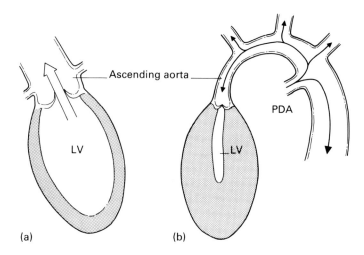

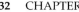

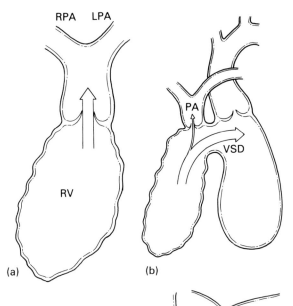

Fig. 3.3.1 (*above*) The relationship
between vessel and chamber
size and blood flow.
(a) Normal heart
(b) aortic atresia. (For
explanation see text.)

Fig. 3.3.2 (*right*)
(a) Normal heart
(b) tetralogy of Fallot.
The small pulmonary
arteries reflect the low
pulmonary flow in a patient
with severe tetralogy of Fallot.

Fig. 3.3.3 (*right*) Atrial septal defect.
Very large pulmonary arteries in atrial
septal defect reflecting increased pulmonary flow.

rection, for example) and other factors — the pressure in the pulmonary arteries in particular — affect pulmonary artery size, so that in some cases we are looking at the situation 'as it was' and not necessarily as it is. But this too may give us helpful information.

Just as vessel size is proportional to blood flow, so too is ventricular size — except in one particular situation; the next example of angiography providing physiological information.

Impaired ventricular function. Just as vessel size is related to the flow through the vessel, so too is the volume of a ventricle proportional to its 'stroke volume' (the volume of blood ejected from the ventricle during each systole). In a normally functioning ventricle the relationship between the volume of the (left) ventricle at 'end-diastole' (LVEDV) and its stroke volume (LVSV) is linear. The stroke volume of a ventricle may include blood passing backwards (as in mitral regurgitation) or blood passing across an intracardiac shunt (as in VSD) as well as the forward stroke volume. However, the total stroke volume can still be calculated, as it is the difference between the volume at end-diastole (LVEDV) and that at end-systole (LVESV). Thus:

LVSV = LVEDV − LVESV

The relationship between LVEDV and LVSV is termed '*the ejection fraction*': .

ejection fraction = LVEDV − LVESV/LVEDV

and is normally around 0.7 or 70% (Fig. 3.4a).

A ventricle that is volume-loaded because of valvar regurgitation or a left-to-right shunt will be large, but provided it is functioning normally it will still have an ejection fraction of 0.7. This is not the case if ventricular systolic function is impaired. Under these circumstances the ejection fraction falls. Such ventricles are easily recognised angiographically; they are large (increased end-diastolic volume) with very little change in volume during the cardiac cycle, since end-systolic volume is much larger in relation to end-diastolic volume than would be the case if the ejection fraction were normal. Patients with a 'dilated cardiomyopathy' have ventricles like this.

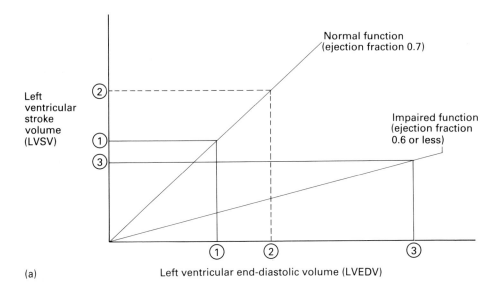

(a)

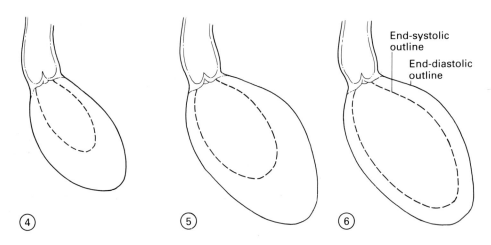

Fig. 3.4 (a) The relationship between ventricular volume and volume load (stroke volume). (1) Normal left ventricular function and stroke volume. (2) Normal left ventricular function with increased volume load due to valvar regurgitation or to a left-to-right shunt. (3) Impaired left ventricular function: the stroke volume is somewhat reduced but the end-diastolic volume is very large. (See text for explanation.) The angiographic appearances of (4) normal left ventricle in systole and diastole. (5) Volume loaded ventricle. (6) Ventricle with impaired function — e.g. dilated cardiomyopathy (*continued opposite*).

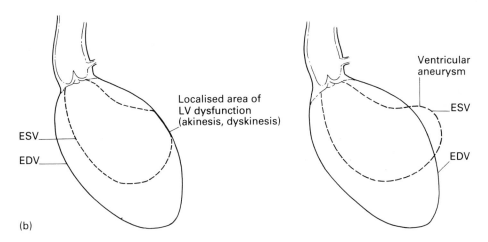

Fig. 3.4 (b) Angiographic appearances of left ventricular dysfunction due to coronary artery disease.

In coronary artery disease there may be areas of the (left) ventricle that are damaged (as by an infarct), while other areas are functioning normally. Such 'patchy' impairment of ventricular function is characteristic of 'ischaemic (coronary) heart disease'. Terms such as 'dyskinesis', 'hypokinesis' and 'akinesis' have been coined to describe various patterns of localised ventricular dysfunction; an area may contract (or relax) asynchronously or its contraction is reduced in amplitude or even absent. If the myocardium has become replaced by fibrous tissue following a previous myocardial infarct the wall of the ventricle may actually bulge outward during systole — a ventricular 'aneurysm'. All these features can be detected by injecting contrast medium into the ventricle — ventriculography (Fig. 3.4b). Ventriculography is an important part of the study of patients with coronary artery disease in order to detect areas of ventricular dysfunction.

Angiographic projections

Cardiologists name projections as though the view obtained was that which they would see if they were looking at the heart from the position occupied by the image intensifier. Thus if the intensifier is directly above the patient's chest, the view is an anteroposterior projection. This is the reverse of the nomenclature adopted by radiologists who refer to the projection in terms of the direction of the X-ray beam — in this case from the source (the tube under the patient's back) to the objective (the image intensifier) so that the view would be a posteroanterior (PA) view. To revert to cardiological nomenclature a 'left oblique' or 'left anterior oblique' (LAO) view is obtained when the intensifier is above the patient and angulated to his left. If in addition the tube and intensifier are angulated in a second plane so that the intensifier is above the patient's left shoulder, the view is from the left and from the patient's head and is termed 'left oblique cranial' (or LAO cranial); angulated towards the patient's feet, the view is 'left oblique caudal' (Fig. 3.5).

Two views are so useful that they have become known by the cardiac anatomy that they best demonstrate. These are the 'four-chamber' and the 'long-axis' views. The four-chamber view has a shallow (25°) left oblique angulation with a steep (45°) cranial angulation. In this view the four cardiac chambers — left and right atrium and left and right ventricle — are separated with minimal overlap; hence the name. The left ventricle has its long axis orientated anteriorly and to the left and this long axis is perpendicular to the X-ray beam when there is steep (75°) left oblique angulation with shallow (25°) cranial angulation.

The projection is chosen to profile the abnormality that is thought to be present. For example, a ventricular septal defect in the inlet portion of the ventricular septum is best profiled in the four-chamber view while one in the membranous portion of the septum is best seen in the long-axis view.

Radiation protection

During fluoroscopy and cine-filming, X-rays are generated and these X-rays are potentially harmful. The patient is only exposed to X-radiation for a short time and on only a few occasions; but the laboratory staff are at risk of exposure on every working day. It is important that laboratory staff recognise this risk and follow certain rules. The most intense radiation is contained within the primary beam and this beam must be 'coned' (e.g. by shutters) so that none of the primary beam is outside the area shown on the television monitor; the operator and assistant(s) must never allow their hands to be seen on the monitor. But the unseen danger comes from 'scattered radiation' — X-rays that have

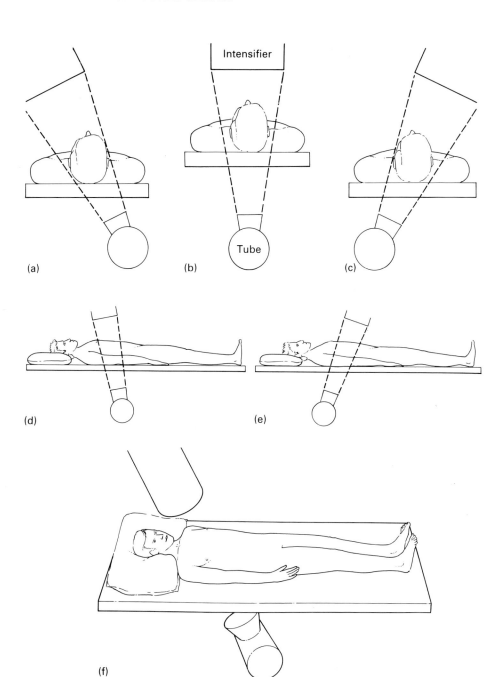

Fig. 3.5 X-ray projections. (a) Left oblique, (b) anteroposterior, (c) right oblique, (d) cranial, (e) caudal, and (f) combined view: left oblique with cranial angulation — e.g. four-chamber view.

passed through the patient and been scattered in all directions by the patient's tissues (Fig. 3.6). We protect ourselves from this scattered radiation by observing these rules:

1 'Lead' aprons must be worn at all times. Those closest to the patient should also wear thyroid shields and, perhaps, protective glasses (the development of cataract is one consequence of radiation of the eyes).

2 Film badges, which record the amount of radiation received by the wearer, must always be worn and checked regularly.

3 Wherever possible protective screens should be arranged around the patient to cut out scattered radiation.

4 No one should be in the procedure room unless needed. The intensity of radiation falls with the *square* of the distance from the source; it follows that merely 'standing back' adds considerably to a person's safety while in the procedure room.

5 No one who is, or might be, pregnant is allowed within the procedure room (nor, except in an emergency, is a patient catheterised who might be pregnant).

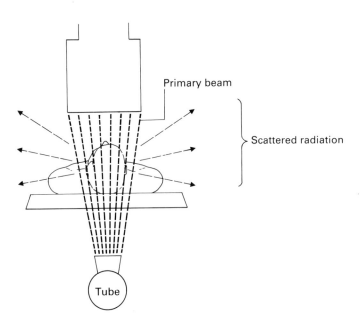

Fig. 3.6 Scattered radiation — a source of radiation exposure for laboratory staff.

6 The operator must remember to use the least possible amount of fluoroscopy — short bursts are all that are needed. Too many operators leave the foot-switch on for long periods.

4 Coronary arteriography

Before 1958 many attempts were made to visualise the coronary arteries angiographically by non-selective (aortic) injections of contrast medium, but it was Mason Sones at the Cleveland Clinic who, in 1958, first obtained coronary arteriograms by injecting contrast medium directly into the coronary arteries — *selective* coronary arteriography. Sones used a brachial arteriotomy and a simple tapered catheter. Subsequently an alternative technique of percutaneous transfemoral coronary arteriography using *preshaped* catheters was developed — notably by Judkins (a radiologist). These two techniques, with some modifications — notably the use of preshaped catheters, such as the 'Castillo' catheter introduced from a brachial arteriotomy — remain the two basic techniques to this day and are often referred to as the 'Sones' and the 'Judkins' techniques, respectively.

There is much, largely pointless, argument about which is the better technique and which has the lower complication rate. In fact all coronary arteriographers should be equally proficient at both techniques; there are patients in whom the approach from the leg is contraindicated and others in whom the brachial approach is contraindicated. The brachial approach, using an arteriotomy that is repaired at the end of the procedure, has one significant advantage: the patients can be studied as day cases and allowed home on the day of the study. Since closure of the femoral entry site used in the percutaneous (Judkins) technique relies on the formation of a 'haemostatic plug', most operators are reluctant to allow the patient to walk about until the next day in case the plug is dislodged and the femoral artery starts to bleed into the tissues.

There has been an explosive increase in the number of coronary arteriograms performed at all centres; in most laboratories this investigation forms most, if not all, of the work load. There are several reasons for this; coronary arteriography has been found to be simple and safe and coronary artery disease is very common. Another important reason for the increased numbers of coronary arteriograms performed is that, with vein and internal mammary artery grafting and coronary angioplasty being shown to provide effective *treatment*, it becomes necessary to have an exact description of the coronary arteries so that treatment can be matched to the disease that is present.

How coronary arteriograms are obtained

Some centres give a light premedication but often no premedication is needed; the only discomfort is a small 'needle prick' for local anaesthesia and the 'warm flush' associated with ventriculography; the procedure can be completed in 10–15 min. If, because of pain or apprehension, the heart rate and blood pressure fall (vasovagal reaction), atropine 0.6–1.2 mg is given intravenously or through the arterial catheter. Heparin in a dose of 0.5–1.0 mg/kg is given to prevent clots forming on the catheter tip and being washed into the coronary arteries. Heparin also prevents clot formation at the brachial arteriotomy site. When a percutaneous transfemoral approach has been used, someone has to press on the puncture site for at least 10 min or until all signs of bleeding have stopped — and the puncture site must be carefully watched on return to the ward.

As a rule, coronary arteriography is preceded by left ventriculography (though some centres leave this investigation to the end). A left ventriculogram is an important part of the study since coronary artery disease can lead to abnormalities of left ventricular function. At one end of the spectrum are left ventricular aneurysms following myocardial infarction, or such severe dysfunction that we refer to the condition as 'ischaemic cardiomyopathy'. At the other end are localised abnormalities of ventricular contraction and relaxation (dyskinesis) or limited areas of non-contractile scarring (akinesis, hypokinesis). Very poor left ventricular function is a contraindication to coronary artery surgery — indeed such surgery will not significantly improve the situation in patients who are more likely to be suffering from breathlessness than angina. Such patients form the largest group of those having heart transplants.

Lesser degrees of left ventricular dysfunction may help in pin-pointing the ischaemic area and may be improved by revascularisation.

Following ventriculography the catheter is changed to one suitable for coronary arteriography; sublingual glyceryl trinitrate is often given at this stage. The new catheter is manipulated into the right or left coronary ostium. This is most easily achieved during fluoroscopy in the left oblique projection since the two coronary arteries arise in a plane that is at right angles to the X-ray beam in this projection. The catheter is connected to a manifold (Fig. 4.1), which allows an assistant to inject a few millilitres of contrast medium (about 6–8 ml for the left coronary, less for the right) and then to return immediately to pressure recording. The appearances are recorded on cine-film; 35 mm cine-film is almost universally used, with filming rates between

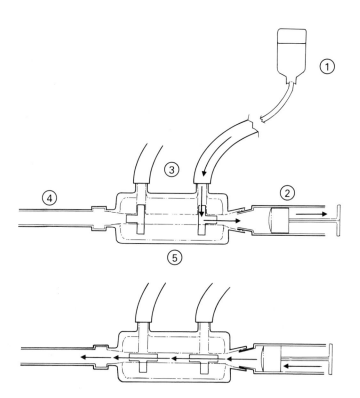

Fig. 4.1 The arrangement used for coronary arteriography. (1) Source of contrast medium. (2) Syringe filled from source of contrast medium. With both taps open to the syringe, 3–10 ml of contrast medium can be injected by an assistant into the coronary artery. (3) Manometer line connected to a pressure transducer. With the tap open to this side-arm and to the catheter the pressure sensed at the catheter tip can be displayed on the oscilloscope. (4) Coronary artery catheter connected to the (disposable) manifold (5) by a rotating luer-lock connection.

25 and 50 f.p.s. Pictures must be taken in multiple projections since the coronary arteries curve around the heart and lesions may be invisible in some projections and well seen in others. The catheter is then manipulated so as to engage the other coronary ostium and the procedure repeated. Electrocardiographic ('T' wave) changes are almost invariable during the injection of contrast medium but, serious dysrhythmias are very rare. Bradycardia is the most common dysrhythmia and the operator may ask the patient to cough so as to restore heart action if asystole is prolonged. Occasionally the catheter may become deeply engaged with a resulting fall or ventricularisation of the pressure displayed from the catheter tip. The recording technician may alert the operator to this potentially risky event.

Although there are only two coronary arteries (left and right; Fig. 4.2), the left coronary artery (LCA) divides almost immediately into two major branches — the 'circumflex' and the 'anterior descending' branches — so that we tend to refer to 'three coronary arteries' or 'three vessel disease'. The anterior descending branch (Fig. 4.3) passes down the front of the heart in the interventricular groove and supplies most of the free wall of the left ventricle and the anterior two-thirds of the interventricular septum. It is a very important artery; if it becomes blocked near its origin, the patient, if he or she survives at all, is likely to suffer severe

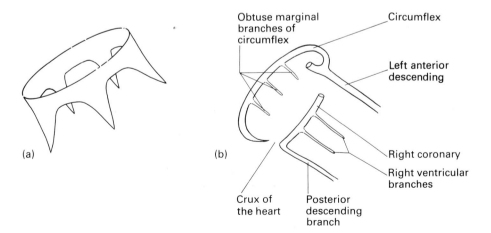

Fig. 4.2 (a) The 'crown' that leads to the term 'coronary'. (b) The coronary arteries.

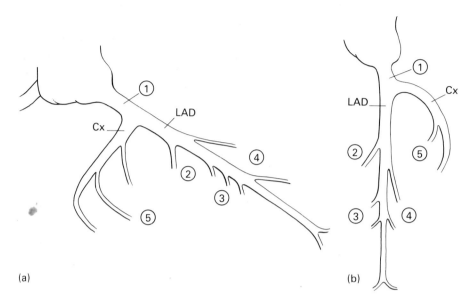

Fig. 4.3 The coronary arteries. (a) The left coronary artery — right oblique projection. (1) Left main stem. (2) First septal branch. (3) Septal branches. (4) Diagonal branches. (5) Obtuse marginal branches. Cx = circumflex. LAD = left anterior descending. (b) The left coronary artery — left oblique projection.

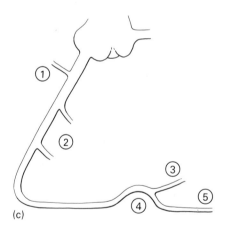

Fig. 4.3 (c) The right coronary artery — right oblique projection. (1) SA node branch. (2) Right ventricular branches. (3) Left ventricular branch. (4) Crux of the heart. (5) Posterior descending branch (in 'right dominant' circulation).

damage to the left ventricle. Proximal stenoses of the anterior descending branch have been termed 'the widow maker'. In addition to septal branches the left anterior descending branch (LAD) gives off 'diagonal branches', which supply the territory between that supplied by the LAD and that supplied by the circumflex branch.

The circumflex left coronary artery (Cx) passes back-wards and to the left, running between the left atrium and the left ventricle until it reaches the posterior interventri-cular groove where its distal branches meet distal branches of the right coronary artery (RCA) which runs forwards and to the right in the anterior atrioventricular groove (Fig. 4.3). In some two-thirds of patients the right coronary artery then supplies the posterior wall of the left ventricle and the posterior third of the ventricular septum by a 'posterior descending' branch — the so-called 'right dominant pattern'. In a small proportion of cases the Cx supplies the posterior descending ('left dominant'), while in the remainder of patients an intermediate pattern is found. Both the Cx and the RCA give off branches at near right angles; those of the Cx supplying the posterior wall of the left ventricle while those of the RCA supply the right ventricle.

Atherosclerotic coronary artery disease (Fig. 4.4) causes the coronaries to become narrowed (stenosed); these stenoses are usually localised and may of course be multiple. Further progression of the disease and clot formation on the atherosclerotic plaque results in vessel occlusion and myocardial infarction. If the disease has been slowly progressive or if the patient survived the heart attack, col-lateral vessels may develop and supply the territory that was supplied by the stenosed or occluded vessel. These collaterals may be from one major artery across to another (e.g. distal branches of an occluded RCA supplied from LCA branches) or between branches of the same vessel. Thus coronary arteriography can reveal a huge variety of patterns of coronary artery disease (Fig. 4.4): we see stenoses and need to describe their severity and position; we see occluded vessels but may see collateral filling of the vessel beyond the site of occlusion; we see the results of vessel occlusion — aneurysms and localised areas of left ventricular dysfunction.

All this information together with the patient's history enables the cardiologist to plan treatment. The most common indication for surgical treatment is when a patient continues to have significant symptoms (angina) despite good medical therapy. In addition there is good evidence that patients with a stenosis of the main stem of the left coronary live longer if treated surgically and some evidence that

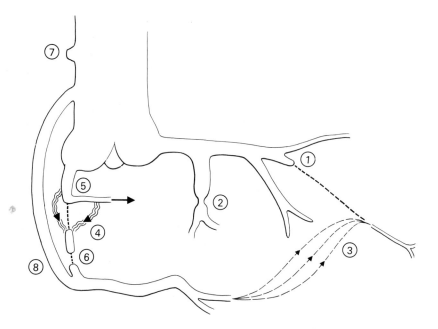

Fig. 4.4 Angiographic findings that may be present in a patient with atherosclerotic coronary artery disease (right oblique projection). (1) A stump of the anterior descending branch of the left coronary artery that has become blocked (occluded) just beyond the origin of a diagonal branch. (2) A concentric stenosis of the main stem of the circumflex branch of the left coronary artery. (3) Intercoronary collaterals that have developed between distal branches of the right coronary artery and the distal segment of the occluded anterior descending branch. (4) Intracoronary anastomoses that have developed between right ventricular branches and the distal right coronary artery, which is occluded proximally (5) just after giving off a right ventricular branch and again more distally (6). (7) The typical appearance of an occluded vein graft — a nipple-like outpouching on the anterior surface of the aorta. (8) A patent vein graft to the right coronary artery.

patients with three vessel and, perhaps, two vessel disease also have a better prognosis if treated surgically than if treated medically. Surgical treatment involves taking a vein from the patient's leg (the saphenous vein) and using it to 'bypass' the stenosis. Lengths of saphenous vein (reversed so that the venous valves do not obstruct flow) are joined to the aorta, proximally, and to the coronary artery, distally, beyond the stenosed segment. An alternative operation is to use the patient's internal mammary artery and anastomose its distal end to the coronary artery (usually the LAD) beyond the stenosis. All this supposes no contraindications to surgery; ventricular function should be reasonably good and the distal vessel must be relatively free of disease. In many cases angioplasty (PTCA) is an alternative way of treating the stenotic lesions and this subject is discussed in Chapter 7.

Unfortunately symptoms may recur following coronary artery bypass surgery — either because of progression of the disease in the native vessels or because grafts have become narrowed or occluded. In this situation coronary arteriography will include cannulation of the grafts so that these may be opacified and studied as well as the native vessels. The technique of graft cannulation is essentially the same as for coronary arteriography; similar catheters are used and multiple views obtained. Grafts are usually inserted on the anterior surface of the aorta; blocked grafts are often revealed by a small nipple-like outpouching of the aortic wall (Fig. 4.4). The internal mammary artery arises from the subclavian artery close to the origin of the vertebral artery and is most easily cannulated when the approach is from the femoral artery.

Myocardial infarction can result in a number of complications, some of which may require investigation by cardiac catheterisation. Left ventricular aneurysm formation is not uncommon and has been referred to already — as has generalised left ventricular dysfunction (ischaemic cardiomyopathy) and heart failure. Occasionally patients who have sustained an infarct involving the ventricular septum develop a ventricular septal defect as the necrotic tissue gives way a few days after the infarct. Such patients present as emergencies with acute heart failure. They need to be distinguished from other patients in whom the infarct has resulted in necrosis and rupture of a papillary muscle leading to acute mitral regurgitation and a similar presentation. In the case of a 'postinfarct VSD', catheterisation will reveal a moderately severe degree of pulmonary hypertension and there will be an increase in oxygen saturation of blood in the right ventricle — a step-up. If a left ventriculogram is performed in the four-chamber or long-axis projection, a defect will be seen in the muscular portion of the ventricular septum. Those with papillary muscle rupture will not have a step-up but a right oblique ventriculogram will demonstrate reflux of contrast medium into the left atrium. Occasionally both conditions can coexist.

Myocardial infarction with scar tissue replacement of the dead myocardium can lead to thrombus forming within the ventricle. This may be detected angiographically but is seldom of clinical importance and embolisation of this thrombotic material is uncommon.

5 Congenital heart disease

Neonates (less than 1 month old), infants and children with congenital heart disease provide some of the most challenging subjects for study in the catheterisation laboratory. There are technical challenges — it may be difficult to introduce the catheters into minute vessels and to manipulate catheters to unusual positions. There are intellectual challenges — the need to make sense of the findings in what may be very complex anomalies and to guide the study appropriately. The patients may be very sick and in a fragile haemodynamic state so that great care must be taken to avoid blood loss, hypoventilation, acidosis, hypoglycaemia and so on. In some laboratories babies are studied with sedation alone; in others general anaesthesia with intubation and controlled ventilation is used. Both approaches have advantages and disadvantages; sedation introduces the risk of undetected hypoventilation and if sedation is too light the difficulty of dealing with a 'moving target'. Anaesthesia avoids these problems but introduces the added risk associated with it.

Every case poses different problems and different questions to be answered but the indications for catheterisation can be listed as:

1 Definition of the basic anatomical abnormality.

2 Measurement of the size of the shunt (if present).

3 Measurement of the severity of valve stenosis (or other obstructing lesion).

4 Measurement of pulmonary vascular resistance.

5 Measurement of pulmonary artery pressure and demonstration of pulmonary arterial anatomy — and the size of the pulmonary arteries.

6 Assessment of ventricular size and function.

7 Elucidation of possible postsurgical complications — occluded shunts, residual defects, and so on.

8 Treatment — e.g. septostomy, valvuloplasty or angioplasty, embolisation.

Of these (and other) indications the demonstration of the basic anatomical derangement, formerly of prime importance, has become an unusual indication since two-dimensional echocardiography has shown itself to be a very reliable way of determining the anatomy. However, echocardiography can only provide indirect information about shunt size, pulmonary vascular resistance, pulmonary artery pressure and valve gradients, and all these measurements may require catheterisation. Some parts of the heart and great arteries are poorly visualised by echocardiography, and angiography may be required to demonstrate aortic arch anatomy (coarctation, interruption) or the anatomy of the pulmonary arterial supply.

Since echocardiography can demonstrate the anatomy, it is common today for catheterisation to be performed not on presentation but months or years later when definitive 'corrective' surgery is being planned. Such patients have often already had palliative surgery (e.g. a shunt) and this may have been done on the basis of the echocardiographic findings alone. This is one reason why emergency studies on neonates are performed less frequently than was the case a few years ago. Another is that prostaglandin can be used to keep the ductus open thus improving arterial saturation while awaiting an elective surgical procedure.

In order to describe the findings at catheterisation in patients with congenital heart disease, we need a classification that recognises broad groups of anomalies. Many such classifications have been proposed; the best is termed 'sequential chamber localisation'. However, a diagnosis such as 'situs ambiguus, double inlet ventricle, double outlet right ventricle' is not only incomplete (though readily completed in a few more lines of text!), but also can only be understood by specialists in paediatric cardiology and not by the majority of 'adult' cardiologists or the students, nurses or technicians to whom this book is addressed. Moreover, although such a description is precise, and unambiguous, the resulting physiological (haemodynamic) disturbance can only be inferred and is not stated. For our purposes, therefore, it may be helpful to have another classification — one based on a haemodynamic grouping of patients with congenital heart disease:

1   Simple left-to-right shunting lesions.
2   Simple right-to-left shunting lesions.
3   Mixing lesions:

(a) with increased pulmonary flow;

(b) with reduced pulmonary flow.

4 Lesions without shunts or with unimportant shunts — valve lesions, coarctation, etc.

5 Impaired myocardial function.

Simple left-to-right shunting lesions

Examples. Atrial septal defect (ASD), partial anomalous pulmonary venous return (PAPVR), ventricular septal defect (VSD), patent ductus arteriosus (PDA), aortopulmonary (AP) window, ruptured sinus of Valsalva, coronary cameral fistula.

Although there are only a few diagnostic possibilities in this group they include some of the most common congenital cardiac defects and are, therefore, of great importance. All are characterised by having separate right and left atria and ventricles and two normally connected great arteries (aorta and pulmonary artery). In all, the resistance to egress of blood from the right ventricle to the pulmonary circulation and the resistance of the pulmonary circulation itself is less than the resistance of the systemic arterial circulation. This is why the shunt is from left-to-right since it is the relative resistances of right and left ventricular outflow that determines the direction of the shunt.

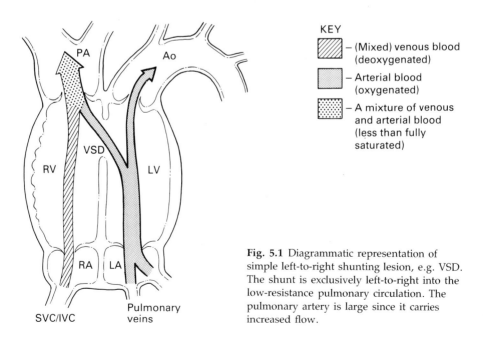

KEY

▨ – (Mixed) venous blood (deoxygenated)

▢ – Arterial blood (oxygenated)

▨ – A mixture of venous and arterial blood (less than fully saturated)

Fig. 5.1 Diagrammatic representation of simple left-to-right shunting lesion, e.g. VSD. The shunt is exclusively left-to-right into the low-resistance pulmonary circulation. The pulmonary artery is large since it carries increased flow.

Simple left-to-right shunting lesion — a typical study. The catheter(s) is introduced into a suitable vein (e.g. the femoral vein) and perhaps an artery. Whether or not a retrograde arterial study is performed will depend on the anticipated anomaly. The venous catheter is then advanced through the right heart to the pulmonary artery (and wedge) while pressure records are obtained at each site. The catheter is then withdrawn through the right heart and great veins while a series of blood samples are taken from each position. This series of samples will reveal an increase in oxygen saturation (step-up) of samples of blood taken from the chamber into which blood from the left heart is escaping. Thus there will be a step-up at atrial level with an atrial septal defect (ASD), at ventricular level with a VSD and so on. The size of the shunt can be calculated using the values for oxygen saturation obtained from pulmonary artery and 'mixed veins' (*see* Chapters 2 and 9).

Information is also obtained from the pressures measured in the right heart; a small VSD for example will have a right ventricular pressure that is less than systemic arterial pressure. A large VSD will cause equalisation of right and left ventricular pressures. Some degree of right ventricular outflow obstruction (e.g. pulmonary stenosis) is possible, but it will not be severe.

Finally, the operator will perform an angiogram to demonstrate the abnormality: selecting the appropriate view, injection site and amount of contrast medium (*see* Chapter 3); for example, in the case of a VSD involving the membranous septum, the injection will be made into the left ventricle, a long-axis view will be selected and 1–1.5 ml/kg of contrast medium will be used. The VSD will be profiled and contrast medium seen to cross to the right ventricle and thence to opacify the pulmonary artery.

Simple right-to-left shunting lesions

These abnormalities differ from the first group only in that the resistance to right ventricular outflow is *greater* than systemic arterial resistance. Again there will be two separate normally connected atria, ventricles and great vessels. The tetralogy of Fallot is the obvious example of this category of congenital heart disease. Others are severe pulmonary stenosis with an ASD and other types of right ventricular outflow tract obstruction (RVOTO). All must have a communication between the right and left heart — as must the first group since without a septal defect or other communication there can be no shunt ('no hole — no shunt').

A subgroup of patients with simple right-to-left shunts are those who started life as group (1) patients, but who have developed pulmonary vascular disease so that pulmonary resistance now exceeds systemic resistance and the shunt has 'reversed' — the so-called Eisenmenger reaction. In a few fortunate patients, shunt reversal is due to the development of increasing right ventricular outflow tract obstruction.

Thus the operator, having demonstrated a right-to-left shunt causing arterial desaturation and having excluded a significant left-to-right shunt, will be concerned to identify the site of the shunt and whether the increased resistance to egress of blood from the right ventricle is due to RVOTO or to pulmonary vascular disease. In the first situation, pulmonary artery pressure will be low and in the second it will be high. Finally, several angiograms will demonstrate

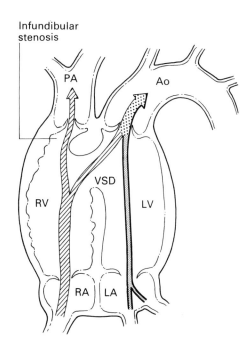

Fig. 5.2 Diagrammatic representation of simple right-to-left shunting lesion, e.g. tetralogy of Fallot. The shunt is exclusively right-to-left away from the high resistance inposed by the infundibular stenosis. The pulmonary artery is small since it carries a reduced flow.

the anatomy; for example in a case of tetralogy of Fallot a right ventriculogram in the right-oblique projection will demonstrate the outflow tract, a left ventriculogram in the long-axis projection will outline the VSD, a pulmonary arteriogram in the four-chamber view will demonstrate the pulmonary arterial anatomy and an aortogram will serve to demonstrate (or exclude) a patent ductus or an anomalous origin of the left coronary artery.

Angiography is often the most important part of the study, since, while the basic diagnosis may not be in doubt, features such as the size of the pulmonary arteries, patency of surgical shunts and number of VSDs may all influence operability.

Mixing lesions

This group of patients includes all those with complex congenital heart disease. All share the feature that pulmonary venous (oxygenated) blood and systemic venous (deoxygenated) blood mix within the heart or great vessels before being distributed to the pulmonary and systemic circulations. Thus all patients exhibit arterial desaturation — the hallmark of a right-to-left shunt — as deoxygenated

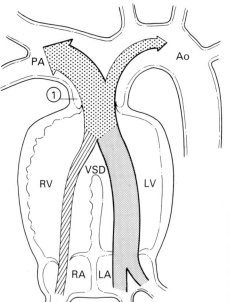

Fig. 5.3 Diagrammatic representation of a mixing lesion, e.g. persistent truncus arteriosus. The two streams mix so that the blood entering the pulmonary artery and the aorta contains a mixture of oxygenated and deoxygenated blood. The pulmonary artery is large since the low-resistance pulmonary circulation accepts a high flow.

blood escapes into the systemic circulation, and all have pulmonary arterial blood of higher saturation than that of mixed venous blood since some fully oxygenated pulmonary venous blood is returning to the pulmonary circulation. Thus there is both a right-to-left and left-to-right shunt. In some patients the pulmonary flow is high, in others it is low as a result of obstruction to pulmonary flow due to sub-pulmonary or pulmonary valve stenosis or atresia. Those with reduced pulmonary flow can resemble closely patients in category (2). How severe the arterial desaturation is will depend on the pulmonary flow (the higher the flow the more oxygenated blood there is to mix with and dilute systemic venous blood). In addition the severity of arterial desaturation is influenced by how completely the two venous returns mix. In complete transposition, for example, mixing can be almost non-existent and the babies are profoundly cyanosed despite having a high pulmonary flow. By contrast patients with persistent truncus arteriosus have both complete mixing and a high pulmonary flow and are only minimally desaturated (cyanosed).

Mixing may be at caval or atrial level (e.g. total anomalous pulmonary venous return, 'common atrium'), or at ventricular and great vessel level (all the many varieties of 'univentricular atrioventricular connection — including tricuspid atresia', persistent truncus arteriosus, pulmonary atresia).

The probability is that the operator will know the basic anatomical diagnosis in advance from two-dimensional echocardiography. However, this may need confirmation at catheterisation, and angiography may be performed to answer questions such as: how many ventricles are there? Is there atrioventricular valve regurgitation? From where is pulmonary flow derived and what is the anatomy and size of the pulmonary arteries? Are there additional unsuspected lesions, such as coarctation or subaortic stenosis? How big are the ventricles and atria and will they support the circulation if corrective surgery is performed? Usually, *physiological* information is also of importance — for example, the pulmonary artery pressure and resistance. Previous surgery may have complicated the situation, while the possibility of further surgery may mean that attempts must be made

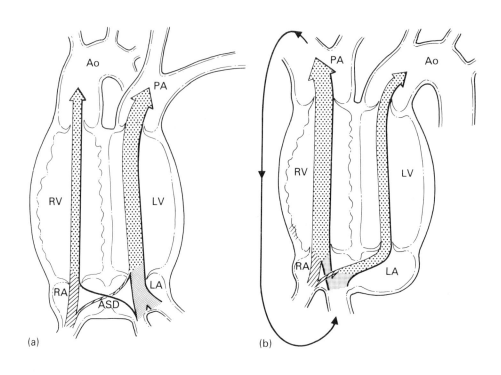

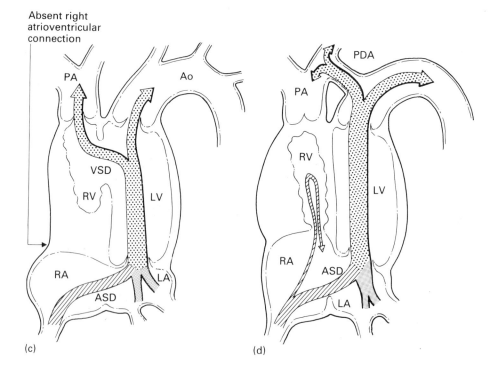

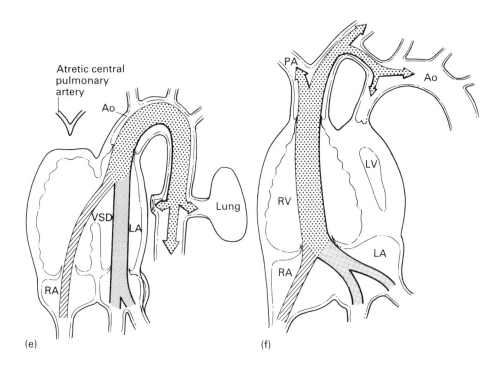

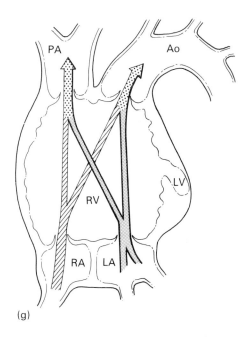

Fig. 5.4 Diagrammatic representation of the central circulation in some of the more common 'complex' congenital cardiac malformations. (a) Complete transposition of the great arteries. Mixing takes place at atrial level. Other possible mixing sites are a VSD and/or a patent ductus. (b) Total anomalous pulmonary venous return. Mixing takes place at atrial level. (c) Tricuspid atresia. (d) Pulmonary atresia with intact ventricular septum. The pulmonary circulation is duct dependent. (e) Pulmonary atresia with VSD. (f) Aortic (and mitral) atresia. The systemic circulation is duct dependent. (g) Common ventricle. This takes many forms. This one is double inlet, double outlet right ventricle — one form of univentricular atrioventricular connection. There may be pulmonary or subpulmonary stenosis — an important determinant of presentation and treatment.

to cannulate the pulmonary artery through a surgical shunt.

The type of angiogram performed will depend on the abnormality present. For example ventriculograms will show how many ventricles there are — and their size. Ventriculography will be needed to demonstrate the presence, size and number of VSD(s) — if present. An aortogram may be needed to reveal the source of the pulmonary blood supply if this is derived wholly or in part from the aorta.

Lesions without shunts — or with unimportant shunts

This group of congenital cardiac defects include: (i) patients with abnormalities that obstruct the flow of blood within the heart or great vessels; (ii) patients with leaking heart valves; and (iii) patients with important malformations of the great vessels or coronary arteries. In category (i) are lesions such as isolated infundibular stenosis, pulmonary mitral and aortic stenosis, cor triatriatum, supravalve mitral stenosis, discrete subaortic stenosis and coarctation. In category (ii) are some uncommon lesions (at least in childhood), such as mitral and aortic regurgitation and Ebstein's anomaly of the tricuspid valve. In category (iii) are some important anomalies, such as aortic atresia and interruption, aortic arch anomalies (including vascular 'ring'), peripheral pulmonary artery stenosis and supravalve aortic stenosis, and anomalous origin of the left coronary artery from the pulmonary artery. I said earlier there may be 'unimportant' shunts and this needs some explanation. In some conditions, aortic atresia for example, there is not only a right-to-left shunt through the ductus but also a left-to-right shunt at atrial level, and these shunts are essential for (brief) survival. Strictly speaking, therefore, aortic atresia is a 'mixing situation'; the important point though is that the presentation is dominated by the severe left heart obstruction and not by the effect of the shunts. In other lesions the effect of the abnormality may be to cause severe ventricular dysfunction — in anomalous origin of the left coronary artery, for example, and this condition might be placed in group (5) with other 'cardiomyopathies'. Inevitably, therefore, this group is something of a 'rag bag' of anomalies.

At catheterisation the operator will be concerned with measuring the severity of a stenotic lesion by obtaining the pressure *gradient* across the valve or other obstructing lesion.

In some instances the operator may proceed to treat the condition, for example by balloon valvuloplasty or co-arctation angioplasty (*see* Chapter 7). For the rest of the conditions it is likely that angiography will provide most of the important information. Angiography will be used to estimate the severity of valve regurgitation and to dem-onstrate the anatomy in conditions such as aortic arch anomalies, coarctation, and so on. Ventricular dysfunction, such as results when the left coronary artery arises from the pulmonary artery and the left ventricle is perfused at low pressure with blood of low saturation, is also assessed angiographically. How this is done is described for the conditions in group (5).

Impaired ventricular function

Normally the left ventricle ejects about 70% of the blood contained within it at each systole. When it has to eject an abnormally large volume of blood we refer to it as being volume loaded. This is the case when there is a large left-to-right shunt or when the aortic or mitral valves are leaking. The ventricle deals with a volume load by dilating so that the volume of blood contained in it at end-diastole is increased. None the less it still ejects 70% of this blood so that the output of the ventricle is increased. We can tell something about the severity of a volume load from the degree of chamber enlargement as visualised angio-graphically. While all this is true of a normally functioning ventricle it is not true if ventricular function is impaired: a poorly functioning ventricle ejects less than 70% of its end-diastolic volume — sometimes as little as 15–20%. Under these circumstances the ventricle is still dilated but there will be very little change in its volume between end-diastole and end-systole when ejection is complete. This is readily apparent from the ventriculogram as described in Chapter 3.

Conditions with a low ejection fraction (dilated cardio-myopathy) are uncommon in childhood; endocardial fibro-elastosis and anomalous coronary origin are two that spring to mind. But there are other forms of heart muscle disease that do not have impaired *systolic* function with a low ejection fraction. In particular, hypertrophic cardio-myopathy can occur in childhood. In this condition there is a gross increase in the thickness of the walls of the ventricle — the septum in particular — and the cavity size is reduced and may be almost obliterated during systole. This can be detected by a ventriculogram — and by echocardiography.

One final group of patients deserves mention — adult patients with congenital heart disease. Such patients may have a relatively benign condition, which has allowed survival into adult life. It may be that the anomaly was not even suspected until some late complication, such as the development of a dysrhythmia, resulted in presentation in middle age. Other patients are those who had a severe lesion but in whom palliative or corrective surgery has allowed survival — and such patients will become increasingly common thanks to advances in the surgical treatment of congenital heart disease.

With the exception of surgical survivors, adults with congenital heart disease usually have a 'simple' anomaly; the most common by far is atrial septal defect. Other conditions that may first present in adult life are VSD, PDA, pulmonary stenosis and aortic valve disease developing on the basis of a congenitally abnormal (e.g. bicuspid) valve.

Several complications may affect patients with long-standing congenital cardiac defects. Of these the most important is the development of pulmonary vascular disease (Eisenmenger reaction). This is especially likely in patients with a large VSD and it is rare for such patients to escape this complication by the time that they are 30 or so years old. But other defects can lead to pulmonary vascular disease, and the measurement of pulmonary arteriolar resistance (see Chapter 2) is a very important part of the study of many adults with congenital heart disease.

Other complications include the development of severe regurgitation at congenitally abnormal heart valves — aortic, mitral (including 'prolapse') and tricuspid. These patients are studied in just the same way as those with rheumatic valve disease (see Chapter 6).

Finally, ventricular dysfunction may result from long-standing congenital heart disease (even after corrective surgery) and supraventricular dysrhythmias are almost invariable in elderly patients. Unfortunately little can be done for patients with ventricular dysfunction, though some may come to cardiac transplantation.

Inevitably this has been a brief review of the way cases of congenital heart disease are investigated in the catheterisation laboratory. There are an enormous number of different congenital cardiac malformations and to describe the findings and plan of investigation in all of them would require a book far larger than this one. But it is this very variety that makes the study of congenital heart disease so fascinating; even the non-specialist must find much of interest in the subject and must learn from these cases a great deal that is helpful in understanding heart disease in general.

6 Valvar and other acquired heart disease

This chapter will discuss a wide variety of conditions that may be studied by cardiac catheterisation; they include diseases of heart valves, diseases of the pulmonary circulation (including pulmonary embolism), diseases of the aorta and diseases of the myocardium and pericardium.

Diseases of heart valves

In the early days of cardiac catheterisation, patients with valvar heart disease formed the bulk of those referred. Rheumatic fever and its consequences were still common, cardiac surgery was largely limited to the treatment of valvar stenosis, and surgery for congenital and ischaemic heart disease was still in its infancy. Today the study of patients with valvar abnormalities forms a relatively small proportion of those referred for cardiac catheterisation. One reason for this is that echocardiography has been shown to be a reliable way of assessing the presence and severity of valvar stenosis and incompetence. None the less some patients are still referred for study; sometimes because the severity of valve disease is in doubt, sometimes simply because coronary arteriography is required to demonstrate or to exclude coexisting coronary artery disease.

A heart valve may be narrowed (stenosed) or may leak (incompetence, regurgitation).

Valvar stenosis. A significantly narrowed (stenosed) valve will impose obstruction to blood flowing across it so that there will be a pressure drop (gradient) between the proximal chamber and the chamber or vessel beyond the stenosed valve. This *gradient* will of course only be present when blood is flowing across the valve; during systole at the aortic and pulmonary valves, during diastole at the mitral and tricuspid valves. Pulmonary stenosis is almost exclusively a congenital defect (*see* Chapter 5) and tricuspid stenosis is uncommon, though small gradients across this valve can be significant.

The *severity* of stenosis is largely assessed by the size of the gradient. This statement requires qualification, however. The variables that govern the magnitude of the gradient are: (i) the volume of blood flowing during each cardiac cycle (i.e. the cardiac output divided by the heart rate); (ii) the time available for blood flow during each cycle (i.e. the proportion of each cycle occupied by diastole — for the mitral valve, or systole — for the aortic valve); and (c) the area of the valve orifice — which is what we want to know. These factors are allowed for in the 'Gorlin' formula, which is used to calculate valve area. Whether or not we employ the Gorlin formula, or one of the simplified forms of the formula described in Chapter 9, it is important to recognise the influence of cardiac output and (to a lesser extent) heart rate on valve gradients. To give an absurd example, there will be no gradient across a valve — however narrowed — if there is no flow! Thus small gradients may be of significance if the output is low — and vice versa. In general we look at *peak systolic gradients* in assessing aortic stenosis and *mean diastolic gradients* in assessing mitral stenosis (*see* Fig. 2.4). A peak systolic gradient of 25 mmHg or more is likely to represent significant aortic stenosis, and a mean diastolic gradient of 10 mmHg or more significant mitral stenosis. The normal mitral valve may exhibit a small gradient in early diastole, but there should be no gradient at end-diastole, so a significant end-diastolic gradient is likely to represent true mitral stenosis.

When studying patients with mitral or aortic stenosis the operator will ensure that the technician is recording the two pressures (proximal and distal to the valve) simultaneously and with the same calibration and baseline. Since a few millimetres of mercury difference is of significance (especially across the mitral and tricuspid valves), calibration will need to be checked for accuracy at this stage. If the valve area is to be calculated the cardiac output will have to be measured at this time.

Two problems remain: (i) it is not always easy to record the two pressures simultaneously; and (ii) it is seldom possible to enter the left atrium in order to record the direct left atrial/left ventricular gradient across the mitral valve. In aortic stenosis it is often sufficient to record the gradient, the pressure drop, as the catheter is withdrawn from the left ventricle to the aorta. In mitral valve disease it is usual to record the gradient between the wedge pressure and the left ventricle. Alternative and more accurate techniques are available. The left atrium can be entered by the transseptal technique (or retrogradely from the left ventricle) and the left ventricle can be entered with the transseptal catheter or directly by transapical needle puncture. Alternative methods of recording aortic gradients are to compare left ventricular and femoral artery pressure or to use a double-lumen catheter.

Finally, it can often be difficult to manipulate a catheter across a stenotic aortic valve; the operator may have to try different catheter and guide-wire combinations.

Mitral stenosis is almost invariably due to rheumatic heart disease; aortic stenosis may be of rheumatic or congenital origin, but calcific aortic stenosis is common in the elderly. The calcium deposits may be easily visible at fluoroscopy.

Valvar incompetence (regurgitation). Almost invariably valvar regurgitation (*see* Fig. 3.2) is assessed angiographically. Radio-opaque contrast medium is injected in the chamber or vessel immediately beyond the suspect valve. If the valve is competent none of this contrast medium will be seen in the upstream chamber. If the valve is leaking it will. Thus if aortic regurgitation is suspected the operator will inject the contrast medium into the aorta just above the valve. If the valve is leaking the contrast medium will be seen to opacify the left ventricle. The rapidity and density of opacification of the ventricle and the readiness with which the contrast medium is washed out are used as indices of severity. Similarly, mitral regurgitation is studied by injecting contrast medium into the left ventricle. An angiographic projection is selected that will profile the suspect valve — the right oblique projection will separate the left atrium from the left ventricle and profile the mitral valve.

There are a number of causes of mitral and aortic regurgitation. Rheumatic heart disease is one possibility but aortic regurgitation can result from abnormalities of the aortic root ('annulo-aortic ectasia', Marfan's syndrome, aortic dissection) and mitral regurgitation may be due to valve prolapse or a 'floppy valve' among other causes.

Secondary effects of valvar heart disease. Valve stenosis or regurgitation will have consequences that are themselves a guide to the severity of valve disease; indeed it is these consequences that cause the patient's symptoms. If a valve is narrowed the pressure upstream will rise in order to overcome the increased resistance to flow. Thus, in mitral stenosis, left atrial and pulmonary vein pressure will rise and as a consequence so will pulmonary artery pressure. Mitral regurgitation will allow left ventricular systolic pressure to be transmitted to a greater or lesser extent to the left atrium. Again pulmonary artery pressure will rise as a result. In both cases the pulmonary arterioles may react to this high pressure so that pulmonary arteriolar resistance may rise in response to a raised left atrial and pulmonary vein pressure. The right ventricle will now face an increased afterload and will hypertrophy. Eventually it may dilate (and finally 'fail') and the tricuspid valve may become incompetent as a result of dilatation of its annulus and its inability to cope with a high right ventricular systolic pressure.

Aortic stenosis imposes an increased afterload (during systole) and will hypertrophy. This results in a 'stiff' ventricle, which fills with increased difficulty so that once again left atrial and pulmonary vein pressure rise. Aortic regurgitation and mitral regurgitation impose a volume load on the left ventricle (*see* Chapters 3 and 5), which will dilate in response. Eventually left ventricular 'failure' may supervene. All these, and other, consequences of valvar heart disease can be detected at cardiac catheterisation and the findings help to build up a picture of the patient's disability.

Diseases of the pulmonary circulation

Many pulmonary arterial anomalies are congenital in origin and some have been discussed in Chapter 5 — as has the development of pulmonary vascular disease (Eisenmenger reaction). But pulmonary vascular disease may also develop as the result of chronic lung disease ('Corpulmonale') or, for no known reason, as an isolated phenomenon, when we call the condition primary (or 'ideopathic') pulmonary hypertension. Catheterisation involves documenting the severity of pulmonary hypertension *and excluding a curable cause*. Thus downstream obstruction (e.g. mitral stenosis) must be excluded by obtaining a normal low wedge or left atrial pressure.

The differential diagnosis of primary pulmonary hypertension includes 'chronic thromboembolic pulmonary hypertension' due, it is thought, to repeated or unresolved pulmonary emboli. The distinction is made by injecting contrast medium into the pulmonary artery — pulmonary arteriography (Figs 6.1 and 6.2). In primary pulmonary hypertension, corpulmonale and the Eisenmenger reaction there are large central pulmonary arteries that taper uniformly and symmetrically. In pulmonary embolic disease the abnormalities are patchy — some areas of lung will be normally perfused while others will have a reduced or absent pulmonary arterial supply.

Pulmonary embolism may also present as an acute emergency. The definitive diagnosis is again made by pulmonary arteriography, which will reveal the emboli as filling defects within the contrast-filled pulmonary arteries. Patients with acute massive pulmonary embolism do not have a very high pulmonary artery pressure — 40–50 mmHg systolic is about as high as is likely to be found — but they

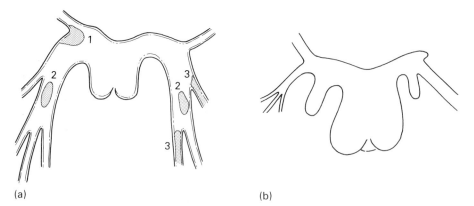

(a) (b)

Fig. 6.1 Pulmonary embolic disease. (a) Recent massive pulmonary embolism. (1) Saddle embolus. (2) Filling defects within the pulmonary arteries. (3) Occluded vessels — cut-offs. The lesions are asymmetrical and the pulmonary artery is not significantly enlarged. (b) Chronic thromboembolic pulmonary hypertension. The pulmonary artery is enlarged and the lesions ('cut-offs') are asymmetrical, but intra-luminal filling defects are no longer seen.

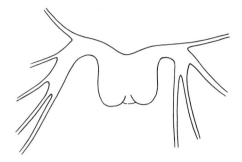

Fig. 6.2 Primary pulmonary hypertension and the Eisenmenger syndrome. Large central pulmonary arteries with reduced calibre of distal vessels ('pruning'). The lesions are symmetrical.

have acute right ventricular failure with a high right ventricular end-diastolic and right atrial pressure.

Diseases of the aorta

Of the acquired diseases of the aorta the classical, but now very rare, example is syphillitic aortitis; a condition that can lead to aneurysm formation and, by affecting the aortic valve, to aortic regurgitation. Aortic aneurysms may also be the result of atherosclerosis, though these more commonly affect the descending thoracic and abdominal aorta than the ascending aorta. Several of the connective tissue diseases may affect the aorta, and one of these — Marfan's disease (syndrome) — affects the ascending aorta and may lead to aortic regurgitation. In Marfan's disease there is striking dilatation of the aorta with an abrupt return to normal calibre before the origin of the aortic arch vessels, so that the aorta resembles a 'Chianti bottle' (Fig. 6.3). Aortic dissection — separation of the layers forming the wall of the aorta — is a feared complication of Marfan's aortitis. Aortic dissection ('dissecting aneurysm') can also occur in atherosclerotic aortas — especially in hypertensive patients — and is an emergency. The dissection may start at the aortic arch and spread downwards or it may affect the ascending aorta, in which case acute aortic regurgitation and rupture into the pericardium are potentially lethal complications (Fig. 6.3). All these diseases of the aorta can be demonstrated by aortography. In aortic dissection the two lumens — the true lumen and the false passage — can be seen separated by a thin radiolucent line formed by the flap of aortic intima. It is important to demonstrate the extent of the dissection, both towards the aortic valve and distally where it may disrupt the origin of the renal arteries causing acute renal failure.

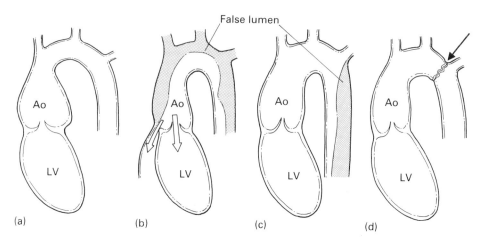

False lumen

Ao

LV

(a)

Ao

LV

(b)

Ao

LV

(c)

Ao

LV

(d)

Fig. 6.3 Some diseases of the aorta. (a) Annulo-aortic ectasia (e.g. Marfan's syndrome). Complications include aortic regurgitation and aortic dissection; (b) and (c) aortic dissection (dissecting aneurysm). (b) Involving the ascending aorta. Complications include tamponade and acute aortic regurgitation. (c) Involving the descending aorta only. (d) Aortic rupture (arrow). Typically follows a car crash — deceleration injury.

Takayasu's disease is another rare condition affecting the aortic arch and arch vessels. Originally described among young Japanese women it is now known to occur in males and in other races. The name 'pulseless disease' is a good one; occlusion of the arch vessels occurs — so that radial and carotid pulses may be absent — and the coronary arteries may also be narrowed at their origins.

Finally, the aorta may rupture. This typically occurs as a result of a sudden deceleration injury as in a car crash (Fig. 6.3). The aorta tears at the point of insertion of the ductus ligament. The victim may survive for a while, but eventual complete rupture is the rule so that it is important to make the diagnosis and to repair the tear. Again these diagnoses are made in the catheterisation laboratory by aortography — the injection of contrast medium into the aorta.

Diseases of the myocardium and pericardium

Four forms of cardiomyopathy are described: dilated (congestive), restrictive, hypertrophic and obliterative cardiomyopathies. Dilated or 'congestive' cardiomyopathy (Fig. 6.4b), in which systolic function is impaired and the ventricle is enlarged with poor contraction and a low ejection fraction, has been described elsewhere (Chapters 3 and 5).

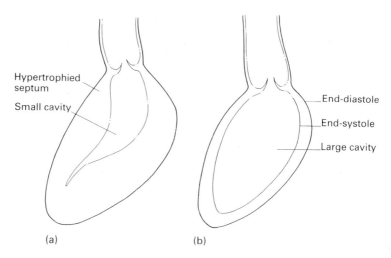

Hypertrophied septum

Small cavity

End-diastole

End-systole

Large cavity

(a)   (b)

Fig. 6.4 (a) Hypertrophic cardiomyopathy (HCM). (b) Congestive cardiomyopathy (COCM).

In 'restrictive cardiomyopathy' the cavity is not enlarged but *diastolic* function is abnormal; the ventricle is stiff and fills with difficulty so that end-diastolic pressure is high. 'Hypertrophic cardiomyopathy' is also primarily a disorder of diastolic function, but it is characterised by gross increase in the thickness of the myocardium — the septum in particular — so that the cavity may be almost obliterated during systole (Fig. 6.4a) and intracavity gradients may be detected ('hypertrophic *obstructive* cardiomyopathy — HOCM'). In HOCM there are abnormalities of the arterial pulse, which has a sharp upstroke and a 'spike and dome' configuration.

Obliterative cardiomyopathy is rare in this country; 'endomyocardial fibroelastosis — EMF in which the ventricular apex is obliterated, is of this type and occurs in West Africa.

Catheterisation in all these conditions will detect the haemodynamic abnormalities, while ventriculography will display the abnormal ventricular morphology and function. In hypertrophic cardiomyopathy the hypertrophied septum, bulging into the cavity of the ventricle, gives the ventriculogram a characteristic shape, which has been likened to a 'bent banana'.

Important diseases of the pericardium that are likely to

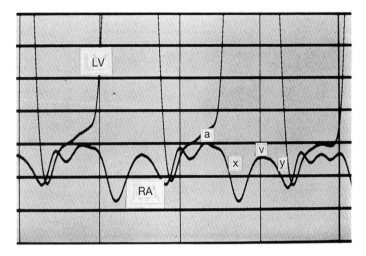

Fig. 6.5 Pressure tracings from a patient with pericardial constriction. Superimposed right atrial (RA) and left ventricular (LV) pressure tracings. Both x and y descents are prominent in the right atrial pressure tracing but the x descent is dominant. There is near equality of the right atrial and left ventricular diastolic pressures (and left and right atrial pressures) suggesting the diagnosis of constriction rather than a restrictive or congestive cardiomyopathy in which left ventricular (and left atrial) diastolic pressures are usually significantly higher than right-sided diastolic pressures.

come to catheterisation are pericardial constriction ('constrictive pericarditis') and pericardial effusion. Pericardial constriction may result as a late complication of inflammation of the pericardium — pericarditis — and tuberculous pericarditis is one such cause. There may be calcification of the pericardium so that the heart is encased in a rim of calcium, which may be easily visible during fluoroscopy. The diagnosis of pericardial constriction is suspected when the filling pressures on the right and left sides of the heart are raised and identical (Fig. 6.5). Thus right atrial and left atrial (or wedge) pressures are the same as are right and left ventricular diastolic pressures. Characteristically the atrial pressure wave exhibits a sharp downward tracing during ventricular systole ('systolic descent'), while the ventricular diastolic pressure has an early diastolic dip followed by an ascent to a plateau during the rest of diastole — the so-called 'square root sign'.

Pericardial effusion and tamponade have similar haemodynamics, but the diagnosis is likely to have been made clinically and by echocardiography; the role of the catheterisation laboratory will be to provide fluoroscopy and haemodynamic monitoring during aspiration of the effusion (*see* Chapter 7).

7 Coronary angioplasty, balloon valvuloplasty and other interventional techniques

Coronary angioplasty (percutaneous transluminal coronary angioplasty — PTCA)

Coronary angioplasty was first performed by Andreas Greuntzig in 1977. Originally it was thought that the procedure would be applicable only to discrete proximal stenoses of a single vessel — and only a small proportion of patients with coronary artery disease have such lesions. Today the indications for PTCA have expanded enormously; in some centres more patients are treated by PTCA than by coronary artery surgery. This has come about partly as a result of increasing experience and skill and partly because of technical developments in the manufacture of sophisticated guide-wires, balloons and catheters.

Patients suitable for PTCA have symptoms (angina) that are poorly controlled by drug treatment — occasionally in certain asymptomatic patients — and lesions that are suitable for angioplasty. 'Suitable' lesions are preferably short and fairly proximal. Concentric stenoses are more readily passed (with the guide-wire) than are eccentric or 'complicated' ones, and calcified lesions respond less well than non-calcified lesions — but even occluded vessels may be reopened. Multiple vessel disease can be treated — not necessarily at one session — but diffusely diseased vessels or long stenosed segments are unsuitable for PTCA. An important use of angioplasty is in the treatment of stenosed vein or internal mammary artery grafts — though the recurrence rate is rather high. A major disadvantage of angioplasty is that about one-third of the lesions recur; however, if this does happen it almost always happens within 3 months and repeat angioplasty can be performed to redilate the stenosis.

When selecting patients for angioplasty it is important to assess the amount of myocardium at risk should the vessel become blocked during PTCA. When the amount of myocardium at risk is small it may not be necessary to arrange for theatre cover. At the other end of the spectrum patients with stenoses of the left main stem coronary artery cannot be treated by PTCA — such patients would be unlikely to survive long enough for emergency coronary

72

artery surgery to be possible if the vessel became occluded during angioplasty. Thus the decision to attempt angioplasty is only reached after careful review of a recent (within 3–6 months) coronary arteriogram; the operator knows in advance the vessel(s) to be dilated and the size of balloon likely to be needed. Balloons should be of the same diameter as the vessel just before and after the stenosis, though preliminary dilatation with a smaller lower profile balloon may be needed if the larger balloon will not pass the lesion.

Percutaneous transluminal coronary angioplasty is usually performed using a percutaneous approach from the right femoral artery. A 9F valved introducing sheath is used to allow a suitable (e.g. right or left Judkins) 8F 'guiding catheter' to be advanced to the coronary ostium. Guiding catheters have a 'soft tip' to avoid damage to the coronary ostium if they have to be deeply engaged to support the guide-wire and balloon catheter. Coronary arteriograms are performed and recorded (digital storage or video-tape or disc) in multiple projections to select the projections that best display the lesion. These stored pictures provide a 'road map' to guide the operator and allow correct positioning of the guide-wire and balloon. A fine (e.g. 0.014″) guide-wire is steered through the stenosis and advanced as far as possible down the distal vessel. Modern guide-wires have good torque control and the tip can be shaped to allow the wire to be steered into the correct vessel (checked by fluoroscopy in at least two projections) and through the stenosis. The balloon catheter is advanced over the guide-wire and centred at the stenosis. An 'indeflator' is used to inflate the sausage-shaped balloon at a known pressure. Inflation may start at 2–3 atm (202–303 kPa) and increase up to about 10 atm (1010 kPa), or until the 'waisting' caused by the stenosis is seen to disappear. There is no need to continue inflation after this has happened. The result can be checked angiographically before removing the guide-wire — it is dangerous to recross a dilated lesion.

In the early days of angioplasty, operators monitored the distal pressure and pressure gradient and aimed for significant gradient reduction. Not all angioplasty catheters in use today allow distal pressure measurement and improved fluoroscopy allows one to use the X-ray appearances

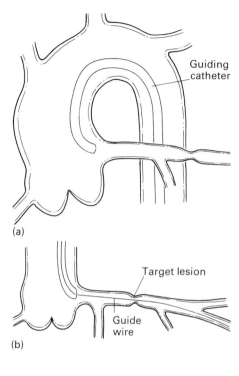

(a)

Guiding catheter

Target lesion

Guide wire

(b)

Angioplasty catheter

Radio-opaque marker

(c)

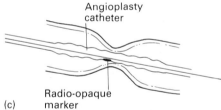

(d)

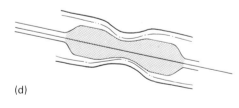

(e)

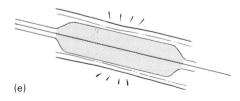

Fig. 7.1 Percutaneous transluminal coronary angioplasty (PTCA). (a) Guiding catheter engaged in coronary ostium. Angiogram performed to show lesion and to provide a 'road map'. (b) Fine (0.014″) guide-wire steered across target lesion and advanced into the distal vessel. (c) Angioplasty catheter advanced until the deflated balloon is centred at the stenosis. (d) Balloon inflated with dilute contrast medium — indentation due to target lesion. (e) Inflation pressure increased until indentation disappears. The procedure is completed by a repeat coronary arteriogram to confirm a satisfactory result.

as a guide to success. However, it is important to monitor arterial pressure (particularly if vasodilators are being given) and to monitor the ECG — either the full 12 leads or leads reflecting the area supplied by the target vessel. S—T changes are likely during balloon inflation, and severe chest pain or the occurrence of ectopic beats is a signal for balloon deflation.

Patients must be heparinised during PTCA and the introducing sheath is left in place until the postangioplasty period is seen to be free of complications and heparinisation can be stopped. Aspirin is given orally before and for several months after the procedure.

The results obtained by PTCA are similar to those obtained by coronary artery surgery; success rates in recent large series approach 90% and mortality is less than 1%. Definitions of success vary but, as with coronary artery surgery, 80—90% of patients experience either complete relief of symptoms or significant improvement in their symptoms. The 20—30% recurrence rate remains the outstanding problem associated with PTCA. Although the mortality is low the incidence of complications is of the order of 5%. The most serious complication that can occur is occlusion of the vessel resulting from dissection or thrombosis at the site of attempted angioplasty, and leading to myocardial infarction. If this happens it may be necessary to transfer the patient as an emergency to the operating theatre for immediate coronary artery bypass surgery. Angioplasty should, therefore, only be performed in a centre with a cardiac surgical unit. It is not always necessary to arrange for a theatre to remain 'on stand-by', but some liason with the surgical team is desirable in the majority of cases.

Balloon valvuloplasty

Catheter-mounted balloons have been in use for a number of years and 'Balloon atrial septostomy' (*see below*) was the first therapeutic procedure to be used in the catheterisation laboratory. However, it was not until 1982 that balloons were used to dilate narrowed heart valves. In that year Jean Kan reported the use of a large catheter-mounted balloon to dilate stenosed pulmonary valves. The technique is so successful and simple that it has now completely replaced surgical valvotomy in patients with 'classical' pulmonary

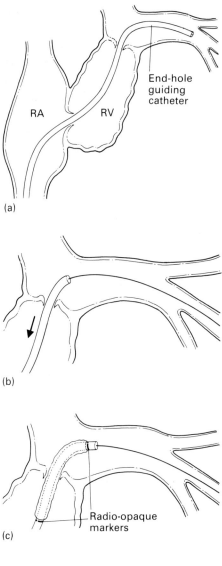

(a)

(b)

(c)

(d)

End-hole
guiding
catheter

RA   RV

Radio-opaque
markers

Fig. 7.2 Balloon pulmonary valvuloplasty. (a)
End-hole guiding catheter advanced from
femoral vein through the right heart to the
left (or right) pulmonary artery. (b) Guide-
wire passed through the guiding catheter to
distal pulmonary artery. Guiding catheter
removed. (c) Balloon valvuloplasty catheter
advanced over the guide-wire and the
deflated balloon centred at the stenotic
pulmonary valve. (d) Balloon (up to 20 mm
diameter) inflated with dilute contrast
medium splits the valve and abolishes the
stenosis.

valve stenosis. Catheterisation is performed percutaneously from the femoral vein, and right ventricular and pulmonary artery pressures are measured. A right ventricular biplane angiogram is performed and the position of the stenosed pulmonary valve noted. Provided the stenosis is of at least moderate severity and the valve is thin (thickened, 'dysplastic' valves do not respond to balloon valvuloplasty), the operator proceeds to valvuloplasty. A long guide-wire is positioned in the right or left pulmonary artery with the help of an end-hole catheter. This catheter is removed (leaving the guide-wire in place) and a balloon catheter threaded over the wire until the deflated balloon is centred on the pulmonary valve. The balloon is then 'inflated' with dilute contrast medium. If everything has been done correctly a narrow 'waist' will be seen in the centre of the balloon; as pressure is increased this waist will be seen to disappear suddenly as the fused valve commisures split open. Repeat pressure measurements should demonstrate a considerable reduction in the gradient across the valve. The balloon has to be chosen with care — its diameter must be about 25% greater than that of the valve ring and it should be as short as possible to avoid damage to the right ventricle or tricuspid valve. Correct positioning of the balloon is important; most failures are due to using too small a balloon or to incorrect positioning of the balloon.

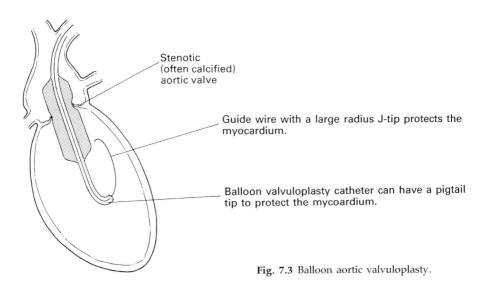

Stenotic
(often calcified)
aortic valve

Guide wire with a large radius J-tip protects the myocardium.

Balloon valvuloplasty catheter can have a pigtail tip to protect the mycoardium.

Fig. 7.3 Balloon aortic valvuloplasty.

The whole procedure can be completed in 20 min or so and the patient can leave hospital the next day. Complications are almost non-existent and restenosis has not been a problem.

Following the success of balloon pulmonary valvuloplasty the same technique has been used to treat aortic, mitral and tricuspid stenosis. Success can be obtained in all these conditions, but the results are unlikely to rival those obtainable surgically. As a result patients selected for the procedure have some contraindication to surgery; elderly patients, patients with severe lung disease or some other condition that would increase the risk of bypass surgery. Elderly patients with calcified aortic valves form one such group, though the success that can be obtained with a balloon is limited and of limited duration — such valves are often so heavily calcified as to respond poorly to stretching by the balloon. Children and adolescents with congenital aortic stenosis form a more promising group; the valves are not calcified and though surgical results are excellent, repeat surgery over the years is likely to be required — with increasing difficulty. Thus valvuloplasty may allow surgical treatment to be postponed.

Balloon aortic valvuloplasty is usually performed percutaneously from the femoral artery. The first difficulty that may be encountered is in crossing the narrowed immobile valve. Once the valve has been crossed a guide-wire with a large diameter J-tip is left in place in the left ventricle and the balloon catheter threaded over the wire and positioned across the valve. As the balloon is inflated its movement becomes quite violent as left ventricular contraction tends to eject the balloon through the valve. Another problem with the technique is that the balloon catheter is large and a large introducing sheath (14F) has to be used to insert it into the femoral artery. Not surprisingly the most common complications are those occurring at the entry site in the femoral artery. Balloons for aortic valvuloplasty should be no larger than the diameter of the aortic annulus.

Balloon mitral valvuloplasty is usually performed using a transseptal technique. Following conventional transseptal catheterisation a guide-wire is placed through the atrial septum, mitral valve and left ventricle and into the aorta with the aid of a balloon-tipped flow-directed catheter. An

8 mm balloon is passed over this wire and used to enlarge the hole in the interatrial septum so that the large (e.g. 25 mm) valvuloplasty balloon catheter can now be passed through the artrial septum and positioned across the mitral valve. Inflation of the large balloon splits the fused mitral commisures and the procedure is completed by a repeat series of haemodynamic measurements. Variations of this technique have been used and it may be necessary to use two balloons, side-by-side across the valve, to obtain a satisfactory result.

Coarctation angioplasty

The use of balloon catheters is not confined to opening narrowed valves; in particular they can be used to dilate narrowed vessels. Thus balloon angioplasty has been used to dilate hypoplastic pulmonary arteries, to relieve stenoses at the site of insertion of 'baffles' used to correct complete transposition and so on. An important use is in treating coarctation of the aorta. Although balloon angioplasty has been successful as the first method of treating 'native' coarctation it is more commonly used to treat recoarctation. By recoarctation we mean a coarctation (narrowed segment of the aorta) that has recurred following surgical treatment — or was not adequately relieved by the original operation.

The technique involves the percutaneous transfemoral (artery) insertion of a balloon catheter over a previously positioned guide-wire. The diameter of the balloon should be no more than that of the aorta above and below the

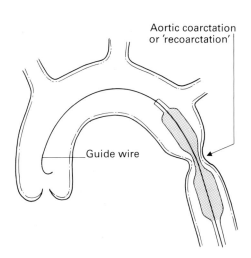

Aortic coarctation or 'recoarctation'

Guide wire

Fig. 7.4 Coarctation angioplasty.

coarctation and the balloon should be as short as possible to avoid damage to the aortic arch, since a curved balloon will tend to straighten during inflation. The result is checked by a repeat aortogram; it is important that following 'aorto-plasty' all catheter exchanges should be made over a guide-wire, which is left in place across the coarctation. There is always a danger of perforating a vessel at the point at which it has been stretched, with inevitable intimal and medial disruption. This is true of both aortic and coronary angioplasty.

Balloon atrial septostomy

This, the first of the interventional techniques, aims to tear a hole in the interatrial septum to allow mixing of right and left atrial blood in babies with complete transposition of the great arteries. In this condition the aorta arises from the right ventricle and the pulmonary artery arises from the left ventricle. As a result systemic venous (desaturated) blood passes from the cavae back into the systemic circulation via the right atrium and ventricle and thence into the aorta. Oxygenated pulmonary venous blood passes, uselessly back into the pulmonary artery after returning to the left atrium and left ventricle. Obviously this situation is incompatible with life and survival depends, precariously, on some mixing of pulmonary and systemic venous blood. Mixing may occur across an atrial septal defect or foramen ovale, across a ventricular septal defect (if there is one) or

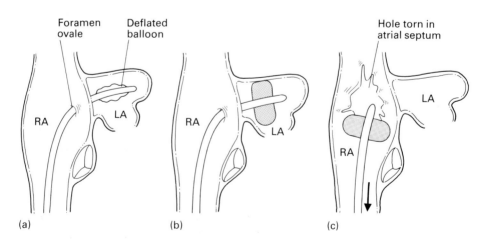

Fig. 7.5 Balloon atrial septostomy (Rashkind).

across the ductus — until it closes. But mixing is often inadequate and these babies present in the first few days of life with profound cyanosis. A palliative operation of atrial septectomy ('Blalock–Hanlon operation') was known to improve the situation, but in 1966 Rashkind and Miller reported the use of a balloon-tipped catheter to achieve the same result without the need for an operation.

The catheter is passed (from the saphenous or femoral vein) across the foramen ovale until its tip lies in the left atrium. The round balloon is then inflated with about 2 ml of dilute contrast medium and then a sharp jerk on the catheter pulls the inflated balloon back through the atrial septum — tearing a hole in it in the process. Rashkind always used to say that success depended 'on the jerk on the end of the catheter!'

Many lives have been saved by this technique; what was an almost invariably fatal condition became survivable — until the baby was around 1 year old when a corrective ('Mustard' or 'Senning') operation could be performed. Today atrial septostomy is not always performed, since many babies are now treated, in the first few days of life by a corrective 'arterial switch' operation.

Occasionally the baby will survive, untreated for a month or so. At this time the atrial septum has become too tough to be torn by a balloon, and another procedure — 'Park-blade septostomy' — may be performed. A special catheter is used in which a small sharp knife blade can be unsheathed when the catheter tip is in the left atrium. The catheter is then withdrawn and the blade slices through the atrial septum.

Other interventional techniques

Just as it is now possible to widen narrowed vessels so too is it possible to close unwanted vessels — all in the catheterisation laboratory. This is achieved by delivering some occluding device or substance into the unwanted vessel. A number of techniques have been used. The simplest is to inject 'Gelfoam' or particles of 'Ivalon sponge' through a precisely positioned end-hole catheter. This technique can only be used if the vessel ends in a capillary network; if there is a large arteriovenous fistula the particles would pass through into the systemic circulation with the risk of cerebral or other embolisation. When there is a large vessel through which small particles would pass, a detachable balloon or 'spring coil' has to be used. Spring coils consist of a coiled length of wire incorporating Dacron fibres. They are supplied within a straight metal cartridge. When extruded from the cartridge they coil up and then resemble a 'woolly bear' caterpillar. An end-hole catheter is positioned with angiographic control within the vessel to be occluded. The spring coil is then pushed from its cartridge directly into the delivery catheter so that it remains straight and can be pushed the length of the catheter by using a guide-wire. As it emerges from the end of the catheter it coils up in the unwanted vessel; clot forms around the dacron fibres and seals the vessel — though several coils may have to be added before occlusion is complete.

Pulmonary arteriovenous fistulae, systemic-to-pulmonary collaterals, anomalous systemic blood vessels to a sequestrated segment of lung and unwanted Blalock shunts have all been treated by this and similar techniques.

When the vessel or communication that is to be closed is large then another technique has to be used. Recently, an umbrella device has been developed for closing a patent ductus arteriosus and, in a few instances, atrial and ventricular septal defects. A special catheter/delivery system is used to deliver the umbrella. This umbrella prosthesis is in fact

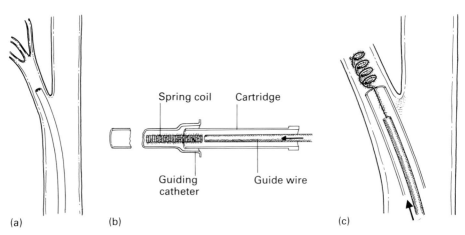

Spring coil   Cartridge

Guiding   Guide wire
catheter

(a)   (b)   (c)

Fig. 7.6 Spring-coil embolisation. (a) Guiding catheter engages (1) unwanted vessel. (b) Guide-wire used to eject spring coil from cartridge into guiding catheter. (c) Guide wire ejects spring coil from guiding catheter and spring coil embolises unwanted vessel.

a double umbrella: each incorporates fine spring-loaded hooks. One umbrella is allowed to open on the aortic side of the duct, the other on the pulmonary artery side.

No doubt other devices will be developed — interventional cardiology may still be in it's infancy!

Pericardial drainage

If fluid or blood accumulates within the pericardial sac in significant quantity the intrapericardial pressure rises and the heart cannot fill. This can be a true emergency — tamponade — or may be a chronic process. One of the most dramatic interventions available to the cardiologist is pericardial aspiration — the removal of this fluid from around the heart. A moribund patient can be restored to normal heart function within minutes as the accumulated pericardial fluid is removed. A needle is inserted, just below the xiphisternum, and advanced upwards, backwards and slightly to the left until the pericardium is entered and fluid can be withdrawn. A guide-wire can be passed through the needle, which is then withdrawn and replaced with a short Teflon pigtail catheter that can be left in place for continued or further removal of fluid.

8 Pacing and electrophysiological studies

by SUE JONES

The natural cardiac rhythm (normal sinus rhythm) originates in the sino-atrial (SA) node — the natural pacemaker — and is conducted by specialised conducting tissue through the atrioventricular (AV) node to the His—Purkinje fibres which then conduct the electrical impulse to the ventricles. Diseases or abnormalities of this specialised conducting system which can result in interruption of the natural rhythm include: abnormal congenital cardiac anatomy, ischaemic heart disease, the result of cardiac surgery, drug therapy and ageing processes causing fibrosis of tissue. Disorders of rhythm which may be life-threatening or cause severe symptoms and impairment of cardiac function may be treated, temporarily or permanently, by therapeutic electrical intervention — cardiac pacing.

The rhythm disorders resulting from these causes and treated by pacing are:

1 Sino-atrial disease (sick sinus syndrome) which may give rise to either severe slowing (bradycardia) of the atrial rate or to tachycardias or to a combination of both.

2 Delays in conduction through the AV node or His—Purkinje system causing complete or intermittent block of the AV sequence or interruption (asystole) of the heart beat. In cases of profound slowing a subsidiary focus, either from the AV junction or from within the ventricles, may take over as the pacemaker but this is not always reliable — hence the need for intervention. Loss of sequential AV contraction is a disadvantage since this is necessary for maintaining the optimum output of blood from the ventricles.

3 Other rhythm disorders which may require pacing are atrial or ventricular tachycardias but these usually require full investigation such as an electrophysiological study (EPS) before the appropriate treatment can be determined.

Cardiac pacing causes the heart to beat in response to an artificial electrical stimulus. A power source (battery) is connected to an often complex electronic circuit which determines timing, output, mode of pacing and so on. The resulting impulse is transmitted to the heart by means of a 'pacing lead' which consists of an insulated conductor and an electrode which may be positioned at any point on the inner (endocardial) or, less commonly, outer (epicardial) surface of the heart.

The site and type of stimulation (pacing) will depend on the rhythm disorder and symptoms that are present. The *modes* of pacing used may be single chamber (atrial or ventricular) or dual chamber (AV — 'physiological pacing'). Any of these combinations may also be linked to a sensor so that the rate of stimulation can respond to situations which require an increase, or decrease, in cardiac output ('rate responsive pacing'). Such systems aim to restore, as far as possible, the natural AV sequential contraction of the heart or its response to physiological demand.

In order to regulate the heart rhythm most effectively the pacing system also needs to respond to/sense any naturally occurring (intrinsic) heart rhythms. This is termed 'demand pacing' and may be applied to any mode of pacing system.

The pacing mode and function is designated by use of a simple international (BPEG & NASPE) position code as described in Fig. 8.1. Pacing systems may be *unipolar* or *bipolar* (Fig. 8.2). Unipolar systems employ a single, *active* electrode in the heart and an earth or *indifferent* electrode remotely placed to complete the electrical circuit via body

BOX	1	2	3
	Chamber(s) paced	**Chamber(s) sensed**	**Response to sensing**
	O = None	**O** = None	**O** = None
	A = Atrium	**A** = Atrium	**T** = Triggered
	V = Ventricle	**V** = Ventricle	**I** = Inhibited
	D = Dual (A + V)	**D** = Dual (A + V)	**D** = Dual (T + I)
	4	**5**	
	Programmability rate modulation	**Antitachyarrhythmia function(s)**	
	O = None	**O** = None	
	P = Simple Programmable	**P** = Pacing (antitachyarrhythmia)	
	M = Multiprogrammable	**S** = Shock	
	C = Communicating	**D** = Dual (P + S)	
	R = Rate modulation		

Fig. 8.1 Code explanation for 'mode of pacing' (boxes 1, 2, 3, 4, and 5).

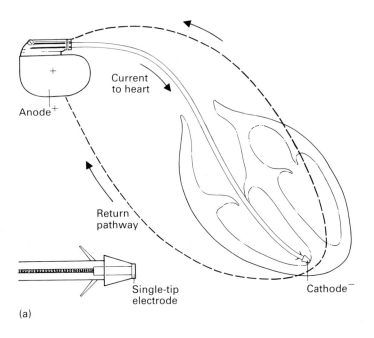

(a)

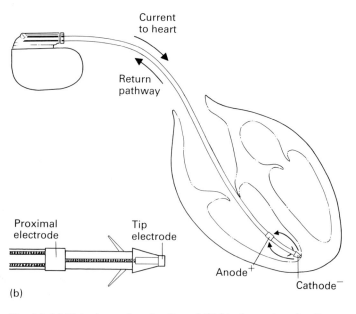

(b)

Fig. 8.2 (a) Unipolar pacing circuit, and (b) bipolar pacing circuit.

tissue and blood. In bipolar systems the two electrodes required are connected by two conductors to the pacing box and both are sited within the heart. Most temporary pacing systems and electrophysiological studies use a bipolar system so as to avoid the need for a second (indifferent) electrode. Permanent pacing systems may be unipolar or bipolar.

Pacing — temporary, permanent or for electrophysiological studies — is usually performed in the catheterisation laboratory as fluoroscopy is needed to precisely position the leads within the heart. The expertise of the same team involved in cardiac catheterisation is needed — particularly technical support personnel for maintenance and use of the sophisticated equipment required for recording and analysing the signals obtained during the procedures.

Temporary pacing
Indications

1   Controlling brady- or tachyarrhythmias.
2   Assessment of a patient's suitability for permanent pacing.
3   Assessment of the system to be implanted for permanent pacing (e.g. choice of physiological or rate responsive system, atrial or ventricular pacing).

Equipment required

1   Pacing leads (atrial and ventricular).
2   Introducers.
3   Pacing pulse generator ('Box').
4   Monitoring/recording equipment.

A bewildering range of equipment is available from a number of manufacturers. Technical reliability is not now a problem as manufacturers are required to meet stringent standards. The choice of equipment therefore depends on specific patient requirements and the preferences of the operator.

The pacing lead

Most temporary pacing systems, whether atrial or ventricular, use bipolar leads. Temporary leads (usually 5F or 6F size) must have adequate stiffness for torque control but must not be too stiff as there is a risk of myocardial perforation.

Ventricular pacing leads are straight or slightly curved to allow the tip to be placed in the apex of the right ventricle. If problems such as anatomical abnormalities are anticipated leads may be used which have a fixation device — screw or flange — at the tip. A few temporary leads have a stylette to stiffen and help guide the lead and such leads may be useful when problems are encountered.

Temporary atrial lead stability is, as yet, an unsolved problem and no currently available lead provides complete reliability. Atrial leads are usually J- or U-shaped to allow positioning in the right atrial appendage or have a loop or flare mechanism to allow some contact against the lateral wall of the atrium. These positions have been found to provide the best signals for sensing atrial activity and for stimulating the atrium.

Temporary AV pacing leads are available in a number of combinations. Hexapolar leads, with two distal ventricular electrodes and four more proximal atrial electrodes, allow the most flexible combination for pacing and sensing but alternatives such as two separate leads or co-axial atrial/ventricular leads are available.

Pacing pulse generator ('pacing box')

For most temporary pacing procedures (excluding electrophysiological studies) a 'pacing box' should have the following characteristics:

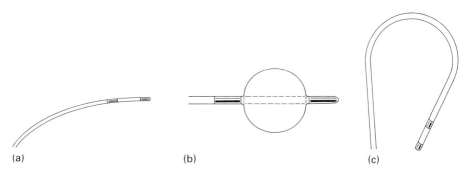

(a) (b) (c)

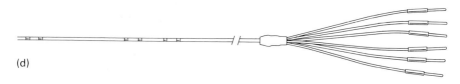

(d)

Fig. 8.3 Some available temporary pacing leads: (a) standard ventricular bipolar; (b) flow-guided balloon pacing lead; (c) atrial J-lead; and (d) hexapolar lead for AV pacing.

1   Mode selection.

2   Rate range: 30–500 b.p.m. (for brady- and tachycardia pacing).

3   Variable output: 0.1–15 V.

4   Variable sensitivity: 0.1–10 mV (suitable for atrial and ventricular signals).

5   Variable AV delay: 50–400 msec.

The controls of the temporary box should be clearly identifiable, easy and safe to operate and the terminal connections should be checked for ease of connection/disconnection of the pacing lead. A lock-on mechanism of some sort with an easy method of uncoupling is recommended for maximum patient safety. A lightweight box is desirable if patients are to be mobilised whilst being paced.

ECG monitoring and recording facilities should be available during all pacing procedures and care must be taken to choose an ECG monitor or recorder that can reproduce the pacing artefact.

Techniques

Temporary pacing leads are usually introduced by a percutaneous (Seldinger) technique. The vein chosen will depend, to some extent, on the procedure to be undertaken. Most therapeutic procedures in which the electrode may be left *in situ* for some time use the right or left subclavian vein as first choice or the internal or external jugular vein if that fails. The femoral vein is occasionally used (e.g. in emergencies).

If temporary atrial leads are to be used an approach using upper body veins usually provides the most stable contact with the atrial wall.

Once the lead has been introduced and a good position confirmed by fluoroscopy the wire is connected to the pacing box and the electrical stimulation threshold is measured. Temporary pacing thresholds of less than 1 V are acceptable provided that the position and threshold are stable. The threshold is measured by initiating stimulation at a rate greater than the patient's intrinsic rate and then reducing the output voltage until capture is lost.

Stability is tested by setting the output to 1 V and encouraging the patient to take deep breaths and to cough and sniff whilst ensuring that capture is maintained during these manoeuvres.

The output setting of the box should be left at a value that provides at least a threefold margin of safety above the threshold. Sensing should be established by ensuring that the pacing box responds to the intrinsic cardiac rhythm (if present) before the lead is secured into place. Connection of the box to the pacing lead may be direct or by means of a connecting cable if more flexibility is required. It is important to ensure that all connections are secure as the patient may be pacing-dependent and, therefore, at risk of asystole if the pacing circuit is interrupted.

Regular checks and maintenance should be carried out on all equipment used for pacing. These checks include:

1   Regular replacement of batteries.
2   Checking output levels.
3   Checking rates.
4   Testing sensing levels.

Complications

The most commonly seen complications are:

1   Displacement of the electrode. With ventricular pacing this may lead to perforation of the ventricular wall with resulting diaphragmatic stimulation or even tamponade. Displacement may also lead to loss of capture or of sensing.
2   Infection. Despite the prophylactic use of antibiotics local infection is not uncommon and may lead to systemic infection.
3   Pneumothorax. This complication can follow subclavian vein puncture.

Permanent cardiac pacing
Indications

The indications for permanent pacing and the choice of system have been documented by many authorities and are internationally accepted (*J. Amer. Coll. Cardiol.* 1984; **4**; 434 and *Circulation* 1984; **70**; 331A). Local considerations which may, nonetheless, influence the choice of system include the funds available, patient age and prognosis, and the availability of support services for follow-up. However the basic requirements for implantation are similar whatever system is to be implanted.

Equipment required

1   Pacing leads.
2   Implantable pulse generator — pacing box.
3   Pacing system analyser.
4   Recorder for intracardiac signals.

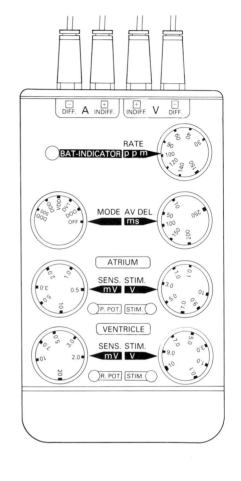

Fig. 8.4 Example of external dual-chamber temporary pacing box.

5 Monitoring requipment.

6 Pacing accessories.

7 Connecting and test cables.

1 Pacing lead

The pacing lead is made up of three components; the conductor, the insulation and the electrode. The conductor transmits the electrical impulse from the generator to the heart and is chosen for its electrical characteristics and mechanical stability. The insulation protects the conductor from body fluid and isolates the electrical signal. The electrode is the heart/lead interface and its shape and size and the material from which it is made is responsible for the efficiency of myocardial depolarisation and of sensing intracardiac signals.

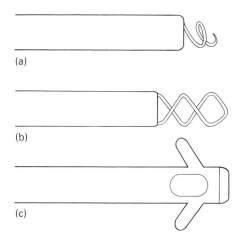

(a)

(b)

(c)

Fig. 8.5 Endocardial lead tip styles: (a) active fixation screw-in type; (b) passive fixation helical coil type; and (c) also passive fixation type but with a tined tip.

As with temporary leads there is a bewildering choice of permanent leads available. Choice depends on the type of system to be implanted (atrial or ventricular), operator-handling preference (flexibility, torque control), size, fixation devices required, anticipation of problems and electrical depolarisation characteristics.

Most permanent pacing leads have a fixation device to provide greater stability of the lead and to avoid the risk of displacement and thus the need for re-operation. Fixation may be 'passive' or 'active'. Passive fixation *assists* contact with the endocardium by means of tines, flanges, helical coils or porous electrodes which allow ingrowth of endocardial tissue. Active fixation involves *aggressive* fixation by the use of a mechanically activated 'screw-in' device. The shape of the lead will depend on the site of pacing; usually J-shaped for atrial pacing and straight or slightly curved for ventricular pacing.

2 Implantable pulse generator ('pacing box')

The choice of permanent pacemaker is determined by specific requirements. The major considerations in selection are typically, size (thin patients and children will need a smaller unit), lifetime of the battery, mode of pacing required, programmability (ability to change pacing parameters such as rate, output, etc.), telemetry or diagnostic functions, and cost. Other factors will be determined by the needs of particular patients — for example some are allergic to certain materials.

Most pacemakers offer a lifetime of approximately 8 years, have a basic range of programmability and are 'physiological' in shape and size. A wide range of pacemakers is on the market and a list of pacemakers and their specifications is available from the British Pacing Group (47 Wimpole Street, London W1M 7DG).

Lead–pacemaker connector compatibility should be verified before implantation as it is only recently that international standards have been agreed and many manufacturer's generators are not compatible with another manufacturer's lead connector.

3 Pacing system analyser

Once the pacing lead(s) is in a suitable position (achieved by fluoroscopy) verification of its electrical stability is required to ensure its long-term reliability and that the threshold and sensed signals are compatible with the pacemaker to be implanted. This is usually done by using an analyser designed specifically for the purpose. Analysers should be chosen to reproduce, as far as a possible, the range of electrical characteristics of the pacemaker to be implanted. In choosing the analyser features should include:

1 Choice of mode.
2 Clear display.
3 Variable pulse output voltage.

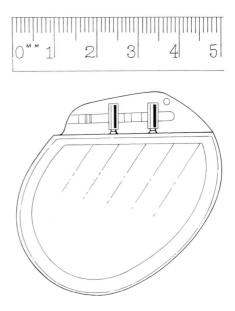

Fig. 8.6 Example of implantable bipolar pacing box.

4 Variable pulse width.
5 Variable rate and sensitivity.
6 Impedance measurement function.
7 Current value read-out.
8 Slew rate.
9 Atrial or ventricular electrogram.
10 Pacemaker test functions.
11 Emergency stand-by pacing.
Pacing system analysers are battery operated and an integral printer or printer output for recording measurements is usually incorporated.

4 Recorder for intracardiac signals

Measurements and recordings of the amplitude and shape of intracardiac signals obtained via the permanent pacing lead are important to determine sensing threshold(s) and thus the sensitivity settings of the implanted pacemaker. A calibrated ECG recorder with suitably isolated input can be used for this purpose and can record bipolar signals by using the standard lead settings I, II and III or unipolar signals by using the V lead connector.

Constant ECG monitoring is needed during pacemaker implantation as it is during any interventional procedure so that suitable monitoring and rescuscitation equipment is also required.

5 Pacing accessories and cables

Permanent pacing procedures may be acute (new implants) or chronic (box or lead changes). In either case, but particularly during box or lead changes, a variety of accessory equipment may be required and must be available. Different screwdrivers for securing the pacemaker-lead connectors, repair kits for broken leads, medical adhesive, lead adaptors for non-compatible leads and connectors, spare stylettes for lead manipulation, connectors and leads for measuring devices and indifferent plates are some that may be required. A range of introducers for different sizes of leads should also be available.

Implant technique

Permanent endocardial pacing techniques vary slightly from centre to centre. Most operators, however, use a cephalic vein approached via an incision through the right or left deltopectoral groove. The pacemaker is implanted subcutaneously in the right or left pectoral region. Two leads

(a)

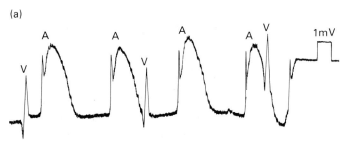

Endocardial atrial electrogram

A = Atrial signal
V = Ventricular signal

(b)

Surface ECG

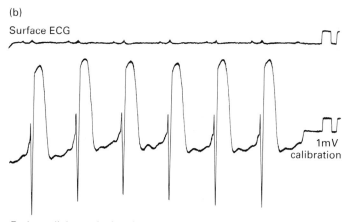

Endocardial ventricular electrogram

Fig. 8.7 Endocardial atrial electrogram. A = atrial signal, and V = ventricular signal. (b) Endocardial ventricular electrogram.

may be introduced into the cephalic vein — if it is large enough — alternatively the cephalic and subclavian vein (entered percutaneously) may be used or both leads can be introduced via the subclavian vein if dual chamber pacing is being performed.* Alternatives to the pectoral site of implantation are a mammary or axillary implant. Right-sided implants are usually chosen in left-handed patients and vice versa.

Once the lead(s) is introduced fluoroscopy is used to

---

* If two leads are being introduced into the same vein leads with a polyurethane coating should be selected as these will not bind against each other — a problem which can lead to difficulties in manipulation.

establish a satisfactory position in either the right atrial appendage (for atrial leads) or, for ventricular leads, the right ventricular apex or outflow tract. Each position is characterised by a typical movement of the lead. An adequate slack, or loop, needs to be left to avoid permanent tension on the lead once it has been tied into position. Once mechanical stability has been established electrical stability needs to be verified.

There are well-documented guide-lines for stimulation and sensing thresholds both for acute and chronic systems. These thresholds are measured by the system analyser. If measurements are not within the accepted guide-lines, attempts must be made to reposition the lead until acceptable values are obtained. The importance of these measurements is that they will determine the settings of the implanted pacemaker. Although programmability allows some leeway this is limited so that initial measurements must allow for this limitation and for changes in pacing and sensing thresholds that occur with time as fibrosis develops around the electrode.

Typical stimulation threshold levels at 0.5 msec pulse duration are:

1   Acute atrial: 0.4–1 V.
2   Chronic atrial: up to 3 V.
3   Acute ventricular: 0.2–0.8 V.
4   Chronic ventricular: up to 3 V.

Both the shape and the amplitude of the electrogram obtained from the atrium or ventricle will give guidance on the adequacy of contact with the endocardium. Acute signals should show characteristic ST or PR segment elevation similar to an injury current pattern if good contact is established. Acceptable signal amplitudes for atrial signals are >1.5 mV and >3.0 mV for ventricular signals.

Impedance measurements, which indicate the total electrical resistance to current flowing in the pacing circuit, should also be measured. This figure is useful for establishing the integrity of the lead — particularly in chronic systems. A very low impedance (<300 ohm) may indicate insulation breakage while a very high impedance (>1000 ohm) may be associated with partial or intermittent conductor fractures. The normal range of impedance values is 300–1000 ohm.

If any of the measurements obtained fall outside the

normal expected range the use of alternative lead positions, pacing modes or lead types should be considered. For example, if an adequate atrial electrogram cannot be achieved an alternative to atrial pacing may have to be considered since a dual-chamber system may rely on atrial sensing for achieving an adequate increase in cardiac output with increasing atrial rates.

Once a satisfactory lead position is established — visually, mechanically and electrically — the lead is connected to the pacing box and a satisfactory pacing and sensing function must be verified. If the patient's rhythm is one that does not activate the pacemaker then the pacemaker should be activated by use of a sterile magnet before closing the pacemaker pocket. If there is any doubt about pacemaker function all relevant measurements should be rechecked.

The role of the technician in these procedures is particularly important as the operator is relying on the measurements obtained by the technician to establish permanent pacing which has to continue for a number of years. Any mistakes in these procedures can jeopardise the integrity of the system.

Electrophysio-logical studies

Electrophysiological studies (EPS) are used to help in the diagnosis and treatment of patients who present with difficult or complex cardiac arrhythmias that are not immediately diagnosable from the surface electrocardiogram. Using special techniques the electrical signals generated from within the specialised conduction tissue of the heart (the intracardiac electrograms) can be recorded and the endocardial surface of the heart can be mapped to precisely locate the origins of numerous rhythm disorders. In addition to recording the electrograms, programmed electrical pulses can be delivered from a stimulator, via the catheters used for recording, to different intracardiac sites. These pulses can be used to initiate and terminate arrhythmias. They can also be used to precisely measure the timing sequences and relationships between different parts of the conduction system during both normal and abnormal rhythms.

Equipment and techniques

Studies may involve simple or complex intracardiac recording from various sites. A variety of multipolar electrode catheters (pacing leads) are available for this and range from bi- to decapolar. For most routine adult studies

6F bi-,tri- or quadripolar catheters are used for paired recording. The electrodes are usually 1 cm or 5 mm apart depending on the precision of recording required. Closer spacing and smaller sized catheters are available but smaller sizes tend to be less easy to handle and have poorer torque control. Catheter size is important as several may be introduced percutaneously into a single vein in order to minimise the discomfort to the patient. The femoral approach is used for most simple studies whilst for more complex studies, where coronary vein mapping is required, both the femoral and subclavian vein are used for introducing the catheters.

A multichannel recorder and oscilloscopic display are required; they must be capable of reproducing the high-frequency components of the intracardiac signals. The recorder should be able to run at speeds of up to 200 mm/sec to allow for accurate interpretation and identification of the signals — particularly during fast rate tachycardias. For complex studies at least eight ECG channels are required with the ability to switch to any of the 12 surface leads so that both the intracardiac signals and the surface ECG can be displayed and compared. If a limited number of channels is available the usual combination chosen is the orthogonal surface leads I, avF, V1 and V6 together with the appropriate intracardiac signals.

The signals are processed and filtered through a switch box and isolated amplifiers with a frequency range of, typically, 40–100 Hz.

A programmed stimulator or pacing box is required to deliver accurately timed pulses at a constant current or voltage to the heart. Various combinations of pulses are used with a minimum of three premature beats after pacing or sensing the spontaneous rhythm.

Since all patients undergoing EPS are at risk of induced or spontaneous, life-threatening, arrhythmias resuscitation equipment and a synchronised defibrillator should be immediately available.

Indications

Sinus node disease
— sick sinus
syndrome

Patients in whom sinus node dysfunction is suspected may require an EPS to confirm the diagnosis. This is done by introducting an electrode catheter into the right atrium and measuring the sinus node recovery time (SNRT) and sino-atrial conduction time (SACT).

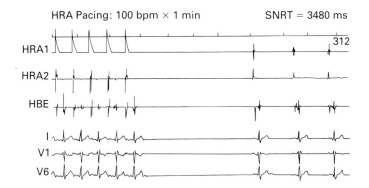

Fig. 8.8 Prolonged sinus mode recovery time (SNRT) in a patient with sino-atrial disease following right atrial pacing at 100 bpm for 1 minute (HRA1 and 2 = high right atrial electrograms; HBE = His bundle electrogram; surface ECG leads I, V1 and V6; paper speed 25 mm/second) (from *Invasive Investigation of the Heart* by G.A.H. Miller, Blackwell Scientific Publications).

Normal sinus node function is supressed by pacing the atrium at higher rates than the sinus rate ('overdriving') for a period of time (usually 1 min) and measuring the time from the last paced beat to the next normal sinus beat after pacing is switched off. Abnormally long recovery times are indicative of sinus node disease. Sino-atrial conduction time is measured by introducing premature atrial paced beats into normal sinus rhythm (or a paced rhythm) and comparing the relationship from sinus to premature beat and premature beat to sinus recovery.

AV conduction assessment

Although the presence of 1st, 2nd or 3rd degree AV block can be detected from the surface ECG it may be necessary to precisely determine the level at which block occurs in order to assess whether, and what type of, pacing may be required. This is done by positioning an electrode catheter across the His bundle in the region of the tricuspid valve and then measuring the conduction time from the atrial signal to the His potential (AH interval) and the time from this His potential to ventricular depolarisation (HV interval). Normal values are AH: 60–110 msec, and HV: 35–55 msec

Since AV conduction abnormalities may only be evident at higher sinus rates, progressively faster atrial pacing rates ('incremental atrial pacing') are used whilst recording the

His electrogram until either natural Wenkebach delay occurs in the AV node (seen as AH prolongation) or abnormal delay is seen by HV prolongation. Abnormal AH prolongation or HV prolongation indicates disease in the conducting tissue.

Supraventricular tachycardias

Patients presenting with supraventricular tachycardias may need an EPS to determine the exact mechanism and location of the arrhythmia. Tachycardias may be due to either abnormal acquired atrial foci (e.g. paroxysmal ectopic atrial tachycardias or atrial fibrillation or flutter) or may arise from re-entry mechanisms through congenitally abnormal accessory (extra) conduction pathways (e.g. atrioventricular pathway in the Wolff–Parkinson–White syndrome, dual intranodal pathways or nodoventricular — Mahaim — pathway). In such cases more complex studies are usually required with recording from multiple sites. Typically electrodes are placed in the high and low right atrium, the His bundle (distal and proximal), the coronary vein (to record left atrial activity) and the right ventricle.

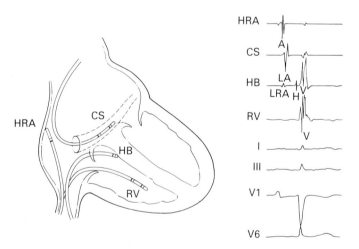

Fig. 8.9 Diagrammatic representation of the heart with electrodes positioned at high right atrium (HRA), adjacent to the His bundle (HB), at the apex of the right ventricle (RV) and in the coronary sinus (CS). Discrete local electrograms from each site are displayed at fast paper speed together with surface leads I, III, VI and V6 (from *Invasive Investigation of the Heart* by G.A.H. Miller, Blackwell Scientific Publications).

Stimulation sequences include incremental atrial and ventricular pacing to assess the antegrade and retrograde conduction properties of the AV node and/or accessory pathways. Stimulation sequences may be used to provide timed ventricular and atrial premature beats during paced and sensed rhythms to assess the refractory properties of the conducting tissue. They may also be used to initiate and terminate the tachycardia being investigated.

Endocardial mapping is performed during the tachycardia to establish the precise location of the accessory pathway.

An important feature of a study of patients with re-entry tachycardias through an accessory pathway is to assess the risk that atrial fibrillation would present since the pathways (unlike the AV node) may conduct very rapid stimuli — thus turning atrial fibrillation into 'ventricular fibrillation'.

Ventricular tachycardia

An EPS may be used to aid diagnosis in patients with suspected, or confirmed, ventricular tachycardia. In the former it may be required to establish the diagnosis when symptoms suggestive of tachycardia exist with no documented surface ECG evidence. In the latter it may be used to evaluate the efficacy of drug treatment or to confirm that the tachycardia is ventricular in origin rather than supraventricular if there is doubt from the surface ECG.

Studies involve delivery of premature stimuli to different sites in the right or left ventricle during normal and paced rhythms. The stimulation protocols, which may vary considerably, attempt to simulate, as closely as possible, spontaneous ventricular ectopic activity at different heart rates. It is usual to deliver up to two premature beats to try to initiate the tachycardia. The use of three or more premature beats has a higher number of false-positive results so that the sensitivity of the study is reduced.

The ventricular tachycardia induced during a study is compared with the clinical tachycardia and must provide a 12-lead surface ECG match in order to be acceptable. Symptoms felt by the patient at the time of the tachycardia initiation are also compared as with the clinical situation.

Right or left ventricular endocardial mapping may be performed during a ventricular tachycardia study to precisely locate the site of the ectopic focus.

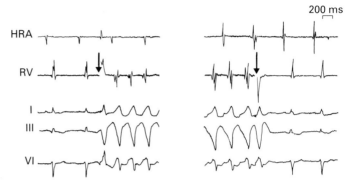

Fig. 8.10 Initiation and termination of sustained ventricular tachycardia by single ventricular premature stimuli. Atrial activity is dissociated both at the onset and termination of the tachycardia (from *Invasive Investigation of the Heart* by G.A.H. Miller, Blackwell Scientific Publications).

Catheter ablation   In cases of tachycardia that are resistant to drug therapy it is sometimes possible to treat the tachycardia by interrupting normal AV conduction (or, occasionally, an accessory pathway) by delivering a high-energy electrical discharge through the catheter. The electrode has to be precisely positioned and, if AV conduction has been interrupted, the patient will normally need to be paced following treatment. This is called 'endocardial catheter ablation'; it is possible to use an ordinary defibrillator as the energy source but specially designed equipment is now becoming available.

This chapter has, inevitably, been a brief review of a complex and fascinating subject; for those — physiological measurement technicians in particular — who become involved in this branch of cardiology there is a wealth of interest to be found. Pacing and electrophysiology are very dependent on advances in technology and these advances have been very great; the field is constantly changing as further technological advance is made. It is not so very long ago that Adams–Stokes attacks were fatal as there was no effective treatment — until the first pacemaker was developed. Today we have techniques for treating most rhythm disturbances — and rhythm disturbances are among the most common disorders of the heart. Untold numbers of patients now benefit from the enormous advances that have been made in this area.

9 Calculations and tables

This chapter explains how to make the calculations that are commonly derived from haemodynamic data obtained during cardiac catheterisation.

Cardiac output —
pulmonary and
systemic flow
The Fick principle

Cardiac output is calculated from measurements of oxygen saturation and from the *oxygen consumption* as described in Chapter 1. For this calculation we need to know or calculate the following:

	Units
Haemoglobin level of the patient's blood	(Hb) gm %
Oxygen capacity of the patient's blood	ml/100 ml
Oxygen saturation of certain samples	%
Oxygen content of these samples	ml/100 ml
Oxygen consumption	ml/min

Oxygen capacity. This is the amount of oxygen that can combine, as oxyhaemoglobin, with 100 ml of the patient's blood when that blood is fully saturated. It does not include oxygen that is in physical solution in the plasma. As a rule this figure is calculated by multiplying the Hb (gm %) by the factor 1.34. Thus, for example, with Hb = 14.0 gm, capacity = 14.0 × 1.34 = 18.76 ml/100 ml.

Oxygen saturation. This is the amount of oxygen bound to haemoglobin in relation to its capacity. Again it does not include oxygen in physical solution in the plasma. Percentage saturation is usually obtained directly by oximetry.

Oxygen content. This is the total amount of oxygen present in a sample of blood (ml/100 ml) and includes both oxygen present as oxyhaemoglobin and oxygen in physical solution in the plasma. It can be measured directly but is usually calculated from the values of oxygen capacity and percentage saturation. Thus:

capacity = 18.76 (ml/100 ml)
percentage saturation = 50%
content = 18.76 × 50/100 = 9.38 (ml/100 ml)

To allow for oxygen in physical solution it is conventional to add:

> 0.3 ml/100 ml where the percentage saturation is above 95%
>
> 0.2 ml/100 ml where the percentage saturation is between 85 and 95%
>
> 0.1 ml/100 ml where the percentage saturation is between 75 and 85%

below 75% saturation there is very little oxygen in physical solution in the plasma; almost all is bound as oxyhaemoglobin.

Oxygen consumption. This is the amount of oxygen taken up by blood passing through the lungs in 1 min. It may be measured but is often simply read from tables of normal values. It is reported in ml/min STPD (standard temperature and pressure, dry). It is assumed that the oxygen taken up in 1 min is in balance with the oxygen used by the body's metabolism so that the figure for oxygen consumption can be used both for the calculation of pulmonary flow (when oxygen is *added* to the blood) and for the calculation of systemic blood flow (when oxygen is *extracted* from the blood).

The calculation. As explained in Chapter 2 the cardiac output, or systemic flow (Q_s), is given by the oxygen consumption divided by the 'arteriovenous oxygen difference':

$$Q_s = \frac{\text{oxygen consumption}}{\text{arterial } O_2 \text{ content } - \text{ mixed venous } O_2 \text{ content}}$$

and the pulmonary flow (Q_p) by:

$$Q_p = \frac{\text{oxygen consumption}}{\text{pulmonary vein } O_2 \text{ content } - \text{ pulmonary artery } O_2 \text{ content}}$$

Example. In a patient with a left-to-right shunt through a VSD the following values were obtained:

Hb	14 gm
pulmonary artery saturation	85%
mixed venous saturation	70%
aortic saturation	96%

pulmonary vein saturation was not
obtained but was assumed to be   97%
oxygen consumption   150 ml/min

Therefore:

oxygen capacity = $14.0 \times 1.34 = 18.76$

pulmonary artery oxygen content = $18.76 \times 85/100 =$
15.95 ml/100 ml (85% of 18.76) but we have to add 0.2
ml/100 ml for dissolved oxygen, so content = 16.15

pulmonary vein oxygen content = $18.76 \times 97/100 =$
18.9 (+ 0.3 for dissolved oxygen) = 18.49

systemic artery oxygen content = $18.76 \times 96/100 = 18.0$
(+ 0.3 for dissolved oxygen) = 18.3

mixed venous blood oxygen content = $18.76 \times 70/100 =$
13.13 (as saturation is less than 75%, nothing needs to
be added for dissolved oxygen)

$$Q_s = \frac{150}{18.3 - 13.13} = \frac{150}{5.17} = 29.01$$

but all values were in ml/100 ml; cardiac output is usually
expressed in l/min, so we have to divide our answer by 10
and obtain a figure of 2.9 l/min.

Similarly

$$Q_p = \frac{150}{18.49 - 16.15} = \frac{150}{2.34} = 64.1 \ (6.4 \ l/min)$$

It is conventional to provide figures for systemic and
pulmonary flow *corrected for body surface area* (BSA). In this
case the body surface area (*see later*) was 1.3 m^2, so the
systemic flow *index* is

$2.9/1.3 = 2.2$ l/min/m^2

and the pulmonary flow index is

$6.4/1.3 = 4.9$ l/min/m^2

If the value for oxygen consumption, on which all the
above calculations depend, was obtained from tables then
it may well be inaccurate (often *very* inaccurate). However,
the ratio of pulmonary to systemic flow (Q_p/Q_s) will be
valid since the same (inaccurate) figure was used in both
calculations. The Q_p/Q_s ratio is, therefore, commonly used
to give an indication of the size of the shunt. In this
example:

$$Q_p/Q_s = 6.4/2.9 = 2.2 \text{ (or } 2.2:1)$$

a moderately large left-to-right shunt.

Indicator dilution/
thermodilution

The general formula for calculating flow from indicator dilution curves is:

$$Q = I/ct$$

where Q = flow, I = amount of indicator injected and ct = the mean concentration, c, of indicator collected over time, t. In practice the calculation is complicated by the need to exclude recirculating indicator and the need to calculate the area under the 'primary curve'. However, thermodilution is the most commonly used 'indicator dilution' method of calculating cardiac output and has the great advantage that the indicator, cold saline, is warmed during passage through the pulmonary circulation so that there is no recirculating indicator to distort the primary curve. The calculations are all performed automatically by a computer, which is an essential component of such 'thermodilution cardiac output' systems.

Shunts

In the example above there was a left-to-right shunt so that pulmonary flow (6.4 l/min) exceeded systemic flow (2.9 l/min). The size of the left-to-right shunt could be expressed simply by subtracting systemic from pulmonary flow:

$$6.4 - 2.9 = 3.5 \text{ l/min}$$

Had the shunt been from right-to-left, so that pulmonary flow was less than systemic flow, we could subtract pulmonary flow from systemic flow and thus calculate the size of the right-to-left shunt in l/min. This method of expressing the size of an intracardiac shunt has two disadvantages. Firstly, the figure obtained is only as accurate as the value used for oxygen consumption. Secondly, there are many patients in whom there is both a left-to-right and a right-to-left shunt (*see* mixing situations, Chapter 5). In these situations, pulmonary flow and systemic flow might be equal so that no shunts would be calculable despite considerable bidirectional shunting. This difficulty can be overcome if we define a left-to-right shunt as that percentage of pulmonary flow that is derived directly from the pulmonary veins (i.e. which has bypassed the systemic circulation). A right-to-left shunt is similarly defined as that percentage of systemic arterial flow that is derived directly from the systemic veins (bypassing the pulmonary circulation). Shunts expressed as percentages in this way can be calculated directly from the relevant values of oxygen saturation, thus:

$$\text{Left-to-right shunt (\%)} = \frac{\text{PA saturation (\%)} - \text{MV saturation (\%)}}{\text{PV saturation (\%)} - \text{MV saturation (\%)}} \times 100$$

$$\text{Right-to-left shunt (\%)} = \frac{\text{PV saturation (\%)} - \text{SA saturation (\%)}}{\text{PV saturation (\%)} - \text{MV saturation (\%)}} \times 100$$

where PA = pulmonary artery, PV = pulmonary vein, SA = systemic artery and MV = mixed veins.

Example. The following values are obtained in a patient with 'complete transposition of the great vessels':

PA saturation = 85%
PV saturation = 97%
SA saturation = 70%
MV saturation = 58%
Left-to-right shunt = 85 − 58/97 − 58 = 0.69 (69%)
Right-to-left shunt = 97 − 70/97 − 58 = 0.69 (69%)

The same calculations can be used to express the percentage shunts when these are pure left-to-right or right-to-left. Thus in our first example of a patient with a VSD the left-to-right shunt is:

85 − 70/97 − 70 = 0.55 (55%)

and the right-to-left shunt is:

97 − 96/97 − 70 = 0.03 (3%)

A small right-to-left shunt is calculated because systemic arterial saturation was 1% less than pulmonary vein saturation.

Mixed venous saturation. If there is no left-to-right shunt the sample of blood taken from the pulmonary artery gives the best estimate of mixed venous saturation — the end result of all the streams of blood of differing saturation and volume that flow into the right atrium. The tricuspid and pulmonary valves and the right ventricle have done the mixing for us! But this will not do if there is a left-to-right shunt causing fully saturated blood to be added to the systemic venous blood. Under these circumstances we have to make an educated guess at mixed venous saturation — based on values for caval and (perhaps) right atrial saturation. Many formulae have been used to provide an estimate of mixed venous saturation. The two most often used are:

(SVC + HIVC + LIVC)/3

or:

[(3 × SVC) + IVC]/4

where SVC = saturation of superior vena caval blood, IVC = saturation of inferior vena caval blood and HIVC and LIVC are samples from 'high' in the IVC (near the hepatic veins and of relatively low saturation) and 'low' in the IVC (near the renal veins and of relatively high saturation), respectively.

'Effective pulmonary flow'. The last of the flow calculations that is sometimes made is the 'effective pulmonary flow'. It is that proportion of the pulmonary blood flow that is effective in taking up oxygen — as opposed to left-to-right shunting blood, which is already fully saturated and, therefore, ineffective in taking up oxygen. Effective pulmonary flow is calculated:

$$\text{Effective } Q_p = \frac{\text{Oxygen consumption}}{\text{PV oxygen content} - \text{MV oxygen content}}$$

Resistances

This subject has also been discussed in Chapter 2. Total pulmonary resistance (R_p) is given by:

R_p = mean PA pressure/Q_p

Pulmonary arteriolar (R_{pa}) resistance is given by:

R_{pa} = mean PA pressure − mean LA pressure/Q_p

where LA = left atrium.
   Sometimes total *systemic* resistance is calculated:

R_s = mean systemic arterial pressure/Q_s

and systemic arteriolar resistance can also be calculated:

R_{sa} = mean systemic arterial pressure − mean right atrial pressure/Q_s

Body surface area This can be calculated from the formula of Dubois:

$$BSA\ (m^2) = 0.007184 \times (weight\ in\ kg \times 0.425) \times (height\ in\ cm \times 0.725)$$

It is more commonly derived from nomograms, such as that provided in Table 9.1.

Table 9.1 Body surface area can be calculated from the height and weight of the patient using the nomogram below constructed according to the formula of Dubois (*Basal metabolism in health and disease*. Lea & Febiger, 1936.)

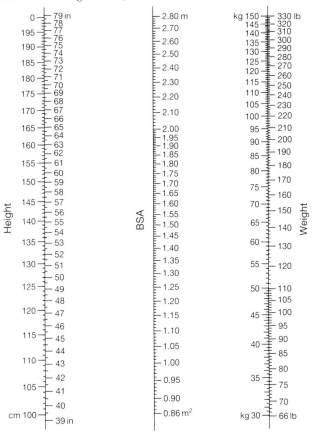

Valve area

The classical formula for calculating the area of a stenotic valve is the Gorlin formula, which takes into account the gradient across the valve, the flow across the valve and the time available for flow to take place. The calculation is tedious but a simplified formula, the 'Hakki formula' gives reasonable results for calculating both mitral and aortic valve areas and has the merit of simplicity. It is:

> valve area = cardiac output in l/min divided by the square root of the pressure gradient (the mean mitral gradient and either the peak systolic gradient or the mean gradient across the aortic valve).

Table 9.2 Oxygen consumption. For children below 3 years of age oxygen consumption is very variable but this table, based on data from Cayler *et al.*, can be used to give an approximation (Cayler, G.G., Rudolph, A.M. & Nadas, A.S. Systemic blood flow in infants and children with and without heart disease. *Pediatrics* 1963; **32**; 186).

BSA (m^2)	Resting O$_2$ consumption (ml/min/m^2)
0.225−0.275	140
0.275−0.325	150
0.325−0.375	172
0.375−0.425	175
0.425−0.475	179
0.475−1.0	174
1.0−1.5	150

Table 9.3 For children above 3 years of age and for adults this table from LaFarge & Miettenen can be used to obtain resting oxygen consumption at varying ages and heart rates (LaFarge, G.G. & Miettenen, O.S.) The estimation of oxygen consumption, *Cardiovasc Res* 1970; **4**; 23).

Age (year)	Heart rate (beats per min)												
	50	60	70	80	90	100	110	120	130	140	150	160	170
Male patients													
3				155	159	163	167	171	175	178	182	186	190
4			149	152	156	160	163	168	171	175	179	182	186
6		141	144	148	151	155	159	162	167	171	179	182	186
8		136	141	145	148	152	156	159	163	167	171	175	178
10	130	134	139	142	146	149	153	157	160	165	169	172	176
12	128	132	136	140	144	147	151	155	158	162	167	170	174
14	127	130	134	137	142	146	149	153	157	160	165	169	172
16	125	129	132	136	141	144	148	152	155	159	162	167	
18	124	127	131	135	139	143	147	150	154	157	161	166	
20	123	126	130	134	137	142	145	149	153	156	160	165	
25	120	124	127	131	135	139	143	147	150	154	157		
30	118	122	125	129	133	136	141	145	148	152	155		
35	116	120	124	127	131	135	139	143	147	150			
40	115	119	122	126	130	133	137	141	145	149			
Female patients													
3				150	153	157	161	165	169	172	176	180	183
4			141	145	149	152	156	159	163	168	171	175	179
6		130	134	137	142	146	149	153	156	160	165	168	172
8		125	129	133	136	141	144	148	152	155	159	163	167
10	118	122	125	129	133	136	141	144	148	152	155	159	163
12	115	119	122	126	130	133	137	141	145	149	152	156	160
14	112	116	120	123	127	131	134	133	143	146	150	153	157
16	109	114	118	121	125	128	132	136	140	144	148	151	
18	107	111	116	119	123	127	130	134	137	142	146	149	
20	106	109	114	118	121	125	128	132	136	140	144	148	
25	102	106	109	114	118	121	125	128	132	136	140		
30	99	103	106	110	115	118	122	125	129	133	136		
35	97	100	104	107	111	116	119	123	127	130			
50	94	98	102	105	109	112	117	121	124	128			

Table 9.4 Normal values for intracardiac pressures.

	mmHg	Range
Right atrium		
'a'	6	1−5
'v'	5	2−8
Mean	3	1−5
Right ventricle		
Systolic	25	15−30
End-diastolic	4	1−8
Pulmonary artery		
Systolic	25	15−30
Diastolic	9	5−12
Mean	15	9−16
Pulmonary arterial wedge (PCW)		
Mean	9	5−13
Left atrium		
'a'	10	4−16
'v'	13	6−21
Mean	8	2−12
Left ventricle		
Systolic	130	90−140
End-diastolic	9	5−12
Aorta		
Systolic	100−140	
Diastolic	60−90	
Mean	70−105	

Index